AARP

New American Diet

Lose Weight, Live Longer

John Whyte, MD

WILEY

John Wiley & Sons, Inc.

Cover image: © nikamata/iStock
Cover design: John Wiley & Sons, Inc.

Illustrations © 2012 by Seth Wise

Published by John Wiley & Sons, Inc., Hoboken, New Jersey
Published simultaneously in Canada

Consult with a physician before starting any diet or exercise program. Information presented is for educational purposes only and not meant as a substitute for the advice of your health care provider.

For general information about our other products and services, please contact our Customer Care Department within the United States at (800) 762-2974, outside the United States at (317) 572-3993 or fax (317) 572-4002.

This and other AARP books are available in print and e-formats at AARP's online bookstore, aarp.org/bookstore, and through local and online bookstores.

Wiley also publishes its books in a variety of electronic formats and by print-on-demand. Some content that appears in standard print versions of this book may not be available in other formats. For more information about Wiley products, visit us at www.wiley.com.

ISBN 978-1-118-18511-7 (cloth); ISBN 978-1-118-22749-7 (ebk);
ISBN 978-1-118-23596-6 (ebk); ISBN 978-1-118-26513-0 (ebk)

Printed in the United States of America

10 9 8 7 6 5 4 3 2 1

Contents

Foreword

by Albert R. Hollenbeck, PhD

This book delivers really good news for your health. Here you'll find a diet that will help you to lose weight and keep it off. With this simple, practical diet, you will be able to live a vital life and may even stave off disease—specifically, heart disease, cancer, and diabetes. The best news is that it works, because it's based on science: the largest study of diet, lifestyle, and health ever conducted in the United States.

The research for this book started twenty-five years ago, when AARP and the National Cancer Institute, part of the National Institutes of Health (NIH), began studying the effects of dietary and lifestyle choices on the incidence of cancer among Americans fifty and older. The study continues to this day, and new data from the study are published in peer-reviewed journals on a regular basis. In the world of scientific research, the joint NIH-AARP Study is in a league of its own for one simple but highly significant reason: it's *huge*, based on more than half a million people. Many similar studies draw conclusions from as few as several hundred participants, concentrating on only a handful of variables.

The size of our sample allows us to draw reliable and specific conclusions about the links among nutrition, health, and longevity. Although no single study can prove anything definitively, this research allows us to settle some long-standing debates about diet and health issues that often leave people confused about what is actually good or bad for them. This study gives us a big picture of what we're eating and how we're living in the real world. It's not just a median or an average; it includes the full gamut of dietary and lifestyle patterns and how they affect our health.

In the world of dietary research, the NIH-AARP Study is exceptional in terms of its validity and comprehensiveness. You've probably read account after account of health news, thinking, "Here they go again!" That's why it was time to write this book: to put it all together in one place to give the general public a one-stop shopping guide to the most current evidence available.

Perhaps the most significant factor about the size of the NIH-AARP Study on which this book is based is that the researchers have been able to look at an extremely broad range of dietary patterns. Smaller studies often lack statistically significant numbers of respondents at a variety of benchmark levels for categories such as fat intake or sugar consumption. The NIH-AARP Study has large numbers of participants across the board, allowing a much more detailed analysis of the effects of dietary patterns than is typically possible.

That's why we can help to clear up the confusion about many things in a field that's become notorious for its less-than-definitive conclusions. What's a person to do when coffee's good for you this week and bad for you next week? Looking at a big sample of the population goes a long way toward eliminating such contradictions. So we answer questions like these: Should you drink coffee? (The short answer is yes, and we tell you how much to drink.) What about red wine? Should you eat red meat, and if so, how much and how often? Fish is good, but is too much harmful? Are white sugars and processed foods taboo? Which fats are the good ones, and which are the bad ones? Do I need a multivitamin? What about other supplements? And how much exercise do I really need? Read on.

So here it is, a mountain of decades of research data about our diet, lifestyle, and health condensed into this very accessible and easy-to-use book. In a way, it's like the discovery of a great new vein of gold. Now, twenty-five years after the study's inception, the resulting riches have become available in the form of hundreds of research papers drawing new, more reliable conclusions about how diet and lifestyle affect health. It's all here for you in *AARP New American Diet*.

Albert R. Hollenbeck is the senior research adviser for AARP and coinvestigator of the NIH-AARP Diet and Health Study.

Preface

"You're fat, and you need to lose weight."

I still recall the surgeon telling that to a patient nearly twenty years ago, when I was a medical student on hospital rounds. The middle-aged woman had just experienced her first heart attack. She was probably about thirty pounds overweight; she was frightened and craved information on how to prevent a second heart attack. What struck me was the fact that the surgeon simply told her what to do and expected results. He gave no information on how to lose weight, and the patient asked no questions. The surgeon didn't discuss what foods to eat and which ones to avoid; nor was there any guidance on when it might be safe to exercise and what exactly the woman should do. I kept thinking, "How can we expect behavior to change without providing the tools to create the change?"

Unfortunately, the patient was back in the hospital six months later, undergoing a triple bypass. Even though we didn't have all the information back then that we do today about lifestyle and disease, we did know they are interrelated. We just did not really do anything about it.

I always wanted to be the type of doctor who would empower patients with information to change their lives. Sure, I would treat disease, but I would also help to prevent disease.

During medical school, I took time to earn a master's of public health to expand my knowledge of how I could improve the lives of populations of people, not just individual patients. I learned about different diseases, but I also learned about medical statistics and study design. I discovered how to analyze the scientific literature and figure out if the study results were actually valid. This training has given me a perspective that has shaped my professional career—I seek a good balance between taking care of the patient in front of me as well patients all over the country.

Throughout my career, I have treated patients with high blood pressure, diabetes, dementia, cancer, and more. Today we have amazing technologies and powerful medicines at our disposal to diagnose and treat disease. The reality, however, is that we also have the ability to prevent and manage many diseases and to live a long healthy life. That doesn't always mean an expensive pill or a fancy test. It's as simple as how we live our lives.

I always talk to patients about lifestyle, and if they are overweight the need to lose excess pounds. Many people are initially surprised, probably because few other doctors take the time to talk about food, stress, physical activity, happiness, and purpose. But I know these are just as powerful as the medicines we prescribe to fight disease. The key is to have the right information to make good decisions.

Writing this book has allowed me to combine my medical skills and public health knowledge with the health communication tools I have learned as Chief Medical Expert at Discovery Channel to give you the crucial information you need in a way you can understand. That's one of the reasons I was so excited to use the NIH-AARP Diet and Health Study as the basis for *AARP New American Diet*. The study represents some of the best published data on how the food we eat affects our health. No other such study has enrolled so many patients over such a long period of time. This research gives us the valuable information we need to lose weight, be healthy, and live longer.

But information has to be understandable. I can have the best message out there, but if no one understands it, it doesn't really matter. People need to hear the message and comprehend it. Sometimes the findings that scientists report and doctors provide can be overly complex. But working with AARP, I have been able to simplify the latest information about diet and health in a way that is practical and easy to understand. It's a real honor to have had this opportunity.

Acknowledgments

"It takes a village." We all have heard that before. In order to write a book it takes a village—and there are some villagers I want to acknowledge.

I want to thank my good friends and colleagues at AARP for thinking of me for this opportunity to work with them on this book. Emilio Pardo is the chief brand officer, and he is always looking for ways to get the best information to the public in a way that is not only educational but also entertaining. I am grateful to Beth Domingo, who initially spoke with me about this project and set everything in motion. Jodi Lipson and her team have been an absolute delight to work with, and they have helped shape the book into a format that works for readers. I am impressed by their commitment to improving the lives of boomers.

Anyone who has written a book knows how vital a good editor is to the process. I have been fortunate to have one of the best in publishing. From the first time I met Tom Miller at a lunch meeting, I knew we would get along well—and indeed we did. He helped me organize my thought processes and distill quite a bit of complicated information into the salient points that readers need to know and can understand. He is the consummate literary professional, and I feel honored that I have had the opportunity to work with him on this book.

I need to thank my mother, who instilled in me early the importance of healthy eating. Mom was always making sure our meals were well balanced while my sisters and I were growing up, and those habits I learned from her have served me well throughout my life. She also has shared with me some secret recipes for her meatballs and other Italian dishes, some of which I've shared in this book!

Finally, I want to express my appreciation to my wife, Alisa, who always gives me encouragement to try different recipes in the kitchen. I must admit she is the better cook, yet she always has a kind word about the meals I create. I'm lucky to have found her, for many reasons, including the fact that we share similar philosophies on healthy eating.

1

The Promise of Weight Loss and a Longer Life

Another diet book? Really? What makes this one different? What am I going to read that's new? I'm sure those thoughts are crossing your mind, and they are good questions.

First, this book is not the typical diet book. I'm using the word *diet* as a noun, not as a verb. What do I mean by that? Too often, people have the mind-set of "I'm dieting" or "I need to diet." But *diet* is not something we do, it's something we live. You might be surprised to hear this, but the smartest and safest diet is actually *no dieting at all* in the traditional sense. This book shows you a diet to live well with rather than a diet for you to "go on."

Too many of us have this idea that we just need to lose ten pounds before an upcoming wedding, a child's graduation, or the start of summer. We deny ourselves all sorts of foods, and when we finally lose the weight, we celebrate it by eating gluttonously and resuming our bad habits. We diet for a few weeks or a few months to reach a short-term goal rather than creating a new relationship with food that we can enjoy for life without even having to think about it. Reading this book will give you a different and fresh perspective as well as a new attitude about food. You'll learn to think about food—your diet—in a completely new way.

Second, what's different and new? After all, hasn't everything about food already been written? Well, actually it hasn't. *AARP New American Diet* provides the most up-to-date information about what you should eat, when you should eat, and how much you should eat in order to lose weight and live longer. It takes the best aspects of the Mediterranean diet and the Standard American Diet (more about that in chapter 3) and blends them into one diet that's realistic and easy to follow. It's not based on one person's beliefs, as some other books are, but rather it is based on the most recent and comprehensive, compelling, well-designed clinical studies from two of the most respected names in health: the National Institutes of Health and AARP. Don't assume that this means the information here applies only to older people—it doesn't. *AARP New American Diet* is for anyone who wants to lose a substantial amount of weight quickly and safely and keep it off as well as live a healthier and longer life and fight disease.

Instead of just quoting studies and giving you references, I'll break the information down for you. I believe that you need useful, credible, practical, and trustworthy information to make smart choices. There's a lot of confusing and sometimes conflicting information out there about what you should eat. This book separates fact from fiction. And since you probably didn't study nutrition science in high school or college, I'm here to give you the important information you need.

What's in it for you? I know you are probably reading this book because you want to lose weight. Taking concrete steps to lose weight is important, and I commend you for that. As a nation, we have been packing on the pounds over the past few decades. In fact, today nearly two-thirds of all adults are overweight or obese—that's roughly two hundred million people and five billion excess pounds. Most Americans are now overweight or obese!

If you're at a healthy weight, you're actually in the minority. I bet you never thought of it that way.

So if you're overweight or obese, you're certainly not alone. But take no comfort in that. Losing weight is hard to do, and getting older doesn't make it any easier. In fact, the longer we've been overweight, the harder it is to lose weight. Our bodies can conspire against us to hold on to the pounds despite our best intentions. That's why you need a proven, scientifically valid method like the AARP New American Diet to lose weight and keep it off—for life!

I am here to help you safely lose weight, but it's equally important for you to become healthier and reduce your risk of getting certain diseases, such as heart disease, diabetes, and cancer. If you already have them, I'm going to try to help you manage them better and maybe even get rid of them.

The promise of weight loss with the AARP New American Diet is not simply a superficial loss of pounds and change in your body shape. It's about something much deeper: filling your body every day with powerful vitamins and other nutrients that have been shown to reduce disease and prolong life. Losing weight is the first step toward becoming healthier, feeling better, staying sharp, staving off disease, and living longer.

Weight puts an extra toll on your body—literally and figuratively—and I want to help you get rid of it. I bet you'd also like to have more energy, think with more clarity, exert more strength, sleep restfully, be in happier moods, and stop suffering from joint pain, indigestion, and lousy cholesterol numbers. Follow the information in this book, and you'll be pleased with the results.

Can weight loss really help you live longer? You bet! What you eat and how much you eat can determine how long you live. Our weight and our longevity are connected. The NIH-AARP Study clearly demonstrated that the food we consume has a big effect on whether we get certain diseases. Some patients have told me that they have had relatives more overweight than they are, and the relatives lived long and seemed to do well. The reality is that these relatives are the exception, not the norm. The number of pounds you carry on your body frame will help determine the quality and quantity of your years—there is no doubt.

More patients than I can remember have told me that their diabetes is not related to their weight: "Dr. Whyte, I've been overweight for twenty years, and I've had diabetes for only two years. You're the first person to tell me my diabetes is related to my weight."

I've got news for you: nearly 90 percent of all cases of type 2 diabetes are related to obesity. Nearly one in three cancers is linked to what we eat and how much we weigh. The NIH-AARP as well as a host of other studies have clearly documented this fact. The harsh reality is that your risk of prematurely dying rises with increasing weight and that this risk increases dramatically by the time you are twenty-five to thirty pounds overweight. You are doubling and tripling your risk of dying by being overweight or obese. Don't shorten your life span by eating the wrong foods! Being overweight increases your chances of developing serious health conditions, including high blood pressure, high cholesterol, diabetes, heart disease, stroke, arthritis, gallstones, incontinence, sleep apnea, and cancer. The good news is that reducing your weight and keeping it off often improves all of these conditions.

Being overweight or obese is associated with not just long-term problems but also with daily struggles. I know many of you would like to breathe a little easier, be more active with your children and your friends, not tire so quickly, have more energy for and interest in sex, and have less pain in your joints. If you can get rid of the extra weight, many times the problems will go away or at least get better. Imagine that you had a thirty-pound boulder strapped on your back or around your stomach and had to carry it around for the rest of your life. You would get used to it over time, but it sure would cause a bunch of problems. It's the same with your excess pounds. Eventually they will catch up to you.

With the AARP New American Diet, I'm going to help you develop a personalized weight-loss plan that ultimately puts you in charge. I'm not going to prescribe every morsel of food you should eat in the course of a day, but I will provide guidelines that are practical and realistic. I'm going to use commonsense principles in helping you lose weight and keep it off. I don't believe in making things complicated, so I'm going to make it very easy for you. I am going to help you get started with 7-day, 14-day, and 30-day weight loss plans complete with meal plans and recipes; there are additional resources at www.AARP.org. I'll even provide you with a grocery list!

By following this diet, you will experience amazing results. What can you expect? The AARP New American Diet will help you to lose weight; reduce your risk of heart disease, diabetes, and cancer; and possibly even prolong your life. You will initially lose a large amount of weight: up to ten pounds in ten days, and probably twenty pounds in the first month if you follow the guidelines.

After the first month, it is going to get more difficult. You'll find out how your body works against you after that initial weight loss and desperately tries to hold on to the pounds. I bet this has happened to you in the past. I'll help you to learn how to over-come these obstacles and not only get to a healthy weight but maintain it as well.

I want you to lose weight, keep it off, and live a healthy life, but I also want you to enjoy food and not deny yourself any food group. Many of you have probably tried different diets with lim-ited, short-term success. That's because a lot of diets work at first, but then real life sets in. The AARP New American Diet is focused on real life: letting you achieve long-term success without gim-micks. I want you to enjoy food—you won't hear me say, "If it tastes delicious or looks succulent, you can't eat it!" There are no fads or gimmicks in this book.

You should be in it for the long haul. You'll need a road map for the journey, and this book provides it. I'm going to help you reprogram the way you think about food. Have you ever seen the TV show *Man v. Food*? In it, the host is challenged to eat an enor-mous amount of food, and he views it as a battle between himself and the plate. This may be similar to your battles, but on a smaller scale (I hope!). You're going to have a few battles along the way in your quest to reach and maintain a healthy weight.

To win the battle, *AARP New American Diet* will give you the information you need to learn more about food and how it affects your body, but it will also teach you how food affects your brain. You'll learn the latest information about the mind-body connection as it relates to diet. Our brains play a powerful role in determining our weight. Our brains and our bodies are wired to send signals about whether we really are hungry, and I'm going to show you how to rewire those signals, because for many of us they have become messed up.

Some foods, especially the high-sugar, high-fat ones we love to eat, can actually be as addictive as drugs. If you are like one of those patients of mine who says, "Sometimes I'm not even hungry, and I'm not even sure why I eat, but I find myself looking in the refrigerator and then chowing down on cold fried chicken, pizza, and ice cream," you won't be, after reading this book.

I'll show you how to get rid of the cravings that sabotage your weight-loss plans time and again. I'll help you to learn that a meal can be enjoyable, tasty, nutritious, and satisfying without you having to feel stuffed; you don't always have to clear your plate, despite what your mother might have told you. The reality is that these are learned behaviors. The best part is that what you've learned, you can unlearn, and instead learn something new. You just need to know how to do it.

The AARP New American Diet does not involve any math— there will be no counting calories or calculating percentages of carbohydrates, protein, and fat. You don't have to weigh your food before you eat it as part of this plan. Calories do matter, and losing weight does involve the number and quality of calories. You do probably need to eat fewer calories as well as better ones, but you don't need to bring a calculator to every meal. You may have done that at one time, and maybe you are doing it now. For most people, it doesn't work, and I want you to think about food in a new way that will last a lifetime.

You'll also learn that although food plays one of the most important roles in how much you weigh and how long you live, there are some other factors involved, such as stress, sleep, physical activity, and even old-fashioned connectivity. I'll give you some simple tips you can incorporate into your daily routine that can help you live longer and keep your brain sharper as well.

As you embark on the AARP New American Diet, I want you to have fun. I want you to be open to new foods, new flavors, new styles of cooking, and new ways of eating. A positive attitude is important: you need to believe you can do this. Picture yourself at your new weight in your new clothes, enjoying food with your family and friends. Maybe you want to wear a pair of favorite jeans that used to fit you and that you've kept around, hoping to be able to wear them again. You can make this happen.

Knowledge is power. This book will finally give you the power to change your body by giving you the best and most reliable information to lose weight and live a healthier life. Let's get started!

2

The Healing Power of Food

Ruth Wants to Keep Her Husband Healthy

"He's scared of having another heart attack," Ruth told me about her husband, John, after his appointment. John is a sixty-two-year-old man with a history of high cholesterol, high blood pressure, arthritis, and heart disease. He's been overweight the entire time I've known him, usually by thirty to forty pounds. He's never lost any weight in between his clinic visits. In fact, he had suffered a heart attack two months before this most recent visit. Ruth always accompanies him to his appointments, and she's not shy about asking the questions she thinks her husband should be asking. I quite like her spunk.

I reviewed all of John's medications: aspirin to prevent clotting, a beta-blocker for blood pressure, a statin for his cholesterol, an anti-inflammatory for his arthritis, and an ACE inhibitor to help with his heart function.

"Have you checked him for diabetes?" Ruth wanted to know.

"Yes, several times. His blood sugars are okay," I responded.

"What about vitamin D?" she asked.

"Yep—checked. It's normal," I replied. "What he really needs to be doing is focusing on losing weight and eating healthier," I reminded her.

John chimed in, "Does that really matter now that I've had a heart attack? Isn't the damage already done? I've never been good at losing weight and am not sure it's worth it at this point."

Ruth glared at him. "He's in a bad mood today," she told me. "Please ignore that question."

Actually, it's a good question, and one I've heard a few times, although I know many more people think it than ask it. I explained to Ruth and John that eating a healthy diet and losing weight works for primary prevention: stopping a heart attack, cancer, or diabetes before they happen. But those lifestyle changes also work for secondary prevention: to prevent another heart attack or control diabetes so it doesn't get worse.

"It's now more important than ever to make changes in your diet," I declared to Ruth and John. "What did you have for dinner last night?" I quizzed them.

"Lasagna," John replied.

"Anything else? A salad? A piece of chicken? Any fruit?" I asked.

"Does apple pie count?" Ruth jokingly asked.

I reviewed the importance of eating food that has carbohydrates, fat, and protein at nearly every meal. Given John's heart disease, I talked about the importance of eating fish as well as of watching sodium content. I emphasized the need for healthy fat.

"Oh, no, Dr. Whyte. He was told he can't eat fat. He has high cholesterol," Ruth insisted.

"That's not quite true, Ruth. He needs to eat healthy fat like nuts," I replied. I proceeded to talk about the different types of fat and why the unsaturated ones are actually part of a healthy and nutritious meal plan. I gave them some handouts that talked about a heart-healthy diet—all the principles of the AARP New American Diet.

Six months later, Ruth and John returned for a follow-up visit. His weight was down almost fifteen pounds, and his blood pressure and cholesterol were normal. What mattered most to both of them was that John had not had any chest pain.

"I'm not sure if it's our new way of eating or just luck, but he's been doing pretty well these past few months," Ruth explained. "He's even talking about starting an exercise program, since his cardiologist said it would be okay."

I told them it probably isn't luck, but rather a combination of his new eating patterns and his prescription medications that is reducing his risk of another heart attack. "Remember, food is medicine. Everything you put in your mouth affects your body," I reminded them.

"I think I believe you now," John said. "I want to be around for my grandkids, so I think twice before I put something in my mouth. We've learned a lot reading the materials you've given us."

Ruth added, "And I've lost five pounds, too, so we're going to keep doing what we're doing."

Two years later, John remained free of any chest pain, and he had lost an additional twenty pounds. I was able to reduce the dosage of both his blood pressure and cholesterol medications.

You Really Are What You Eat

"You are what you eat." I bet you've heard that before. Well, it's basically true.

What we choose to eat ultimately affects how we look, how we feel, and most likely how and when we die. The good news is that you can largely control your mood, your shape, and possibly how long you live and the quality of your life by what you put in your mouth. You're not powerless over how much you weigh; you can be in control of it.

Treat your food like medicine. Do you want to use medicines that improve your life, or do you want to take medicines that cause problems? Like a prescription medication, food can affect every system of your body: musculoskeletal, urinary, endocrine, nervous, digestive, and especially cardiovascular. Putting it in simpler terms, the food you eat affects your skin, hair, bones, joints, brain, blood vessels, heart, stomach, bowels, bladder, and nerve endings. When I phrase it that way, it makes you want to think twice about what you put in your mouth, doesn't it?

Most of us don't eat the right foods. By the "right" foods, I mean food that is nutritious, satisfying, and satiating but also packed with vitamins and minerals to help us live healthy lives. Most of us are eating the wrong things, and too much of them: red meat, processed lunch meats, high-fat dairy products, refined grains and other starchy foods (white bread, white rice, white pasta, white potatoes), processed foods, and sugary and salty snacks. And we drink way too many beverages loaded with sugar.

Instead, we should be eating more fish, lean meats, whole grains, nuts, low-fat dairy, fresh fruit, and fresh vegetables. These are the foods that, according to documented scientific evidence in the NIH-AARP Diet and Health Study, cause weight loss, reduce the likelihood of certain diseases, and prolong life. And we should be drinking much more water.

People are always looking for a magic pill that will make them lose weight and live longer. There is no pill that will do this, but some powerful foods, when eaten at the right times and in the right amounts, can do that. These are the foods that the AARP New American Diet incorporates into its meal plans and recipes.

A good friend of mine who is a dietitian once said to me, "Food is medicine for the body and the soul." She was right.

Food doesn't just affect the way we look; it also directly affects how we think and live.

Three Things to Think About

As we embark on this new journey to healthy eating and longevity, I'd like you to do three things:

1. Stop kidding yourself about what you should and shouldn't eat.
2. Cut through the clutter of information out there.
3. Begin the process of real change.

Stop Kidding Yourself

I'm a firm believer that if you change your attitude, you can change your body. You know deep down that you can't eat cookies and ice cream every day and expect to lose weight. If you're a couch potato watching TV and eating chips most evenings, you know that's not a way to lose weight, either. I don't need to tell you that. And you can't keep saying, "I'll start next week."

There are some basic principles about food that we all know but just simply ignore. I see too many people who keep doing the same bad behaviors and convince themselves that they'll lose weight anyway. Others simply say, "I have the fat gene" and tell themselves that there's nothing they can do about it.

Please stop kidding yourself. You need to admit to yourself that your attitude toward food is wrong and your current plan is not working. You are capable of losing weight and keeping it off, if you use the right tools to change certain behaviors.

Cut through the Clutter

We all read and hear a lot of confusing information about food in the media. One day you hear a report that drinking coffee is good; the next day, a new study claims that drinking coffee will give you a heart attack. One study says chocolate is good for you, but then a month later you're told it might cause a stroke. Is pasta okay to eat, or is it the enemy? We hear wine is okay to drink for dinner and then hear that we should eliminate alcohol completely from our diet.

I get frustrated, and I'm sure you do, too. I can see why you would throw up your hands in exasperation and say, "Why bother?" Between the conflicting and confusing information and the often misleading marketing by food manufacturers, it's hard to know what to do to eat healthily and lose weight. Whom do you believe? Many patients have told me they thought fat-free was healthy, only to learn from me that fat-free products are often loaded with sugar. Or they start eating yogurt as part of their goal to start the day with a healthy breakfast, and then they find out that some yogurts have as much sugar as a Snickers bar (that's probably why I like vanilla yogurt so much!). And is diet soda actually making you gain weight?

Arm yourself with the correct information for a successful weight-loss plan. You've taken the first step toward that by reading this book. Kudos to you! With the knowledge I will give you, you will be in charge of changing your body and improving your health.

Begin the Process of Real Change

Plus ça change, plus c'est la même chose. This French saying means the more things change, the more they stay the same. In terms of healthy eating and maintaining a healthy weight, the French actually do a pretty good job.

Too often we say we're making changes, but we really don't make any real change. Maybe you convinced yourself that you're going to start exercising, but you end up doing it only once a week for fifteen minutes, and then after two weeks you quit. You really haven't changed anything. Or perhaps you decide you're going to start eating a salad for lunch, but then you decide it's too hard to prepare it the night before, or there doesn't seem to be anywhere to store perishable food where you work. So you say you're changing bad habits, but you haven't really made any change. Or worse, you merely exchange one bad habit for another.

You're not alone—80 percent of us give up on weight-loss efforts within five days. We don't even last a week. The key here is for you to embrace a change in the way you eat that you can sustain for life, that will become your new way of eating. It'll become so natural that you won't need to think about it.

There are many different reasons each of us desires to lose weight. It's not an easy process, and there are going to be several false starts, as you've probably already experienced. But when you stop kidding yourself and cut through the clutter, you will be able to make real change.

Fad Diets and Why They Fail

I bet you have tried a bunch of different diets before reading this book. Nearly every one of us has tried two or three at some point in our lives. And every year, at least five new ones come out, promising weight loss with little effort. The problem with these diets is that they are not realistic and don't focus on how we eat in real life. Almost all of them involve denying yourself an entire class of food, such as fat or carbohydrates. One even says you mustn't take the elevator on Thursdays! Others involve complicated food plans and high-level math in calculating the components of what you eat. They all seem to have a gimmick, and most are based on little data to support their advice.

I understand that it sounds sensible, at first, to eat like our prehistoric ancestors did, since they were all of normal weight and didn't die of heart disease and cancer. But when you think about it, does it really make sense? Really? Our lives are vastly different from their lives thousands, if not millions, of years ago, and most people died before they turned forty. You can't expect to adopt habits from a time of life that doesn't apply at all today. Stop kidding yourself—it can't be a good thing to eat red meat all the time. The NIH-AARP Study has repeatedly shown the negative impact that consumption of red meat can have on our health.

Fad diets haven't worked for most people in the long run. Why? Remember, I'm using *diet* as a noun, not a verb. Following the best diet doesn't mean eliminating entire categories of foods. Diets that severely restrict calories or the types of food allowed can lead you to be deficient in the nutrients your body needs to function at its peak. One of the biggest misconceptions is that you need to completely eliminate fat from your diet, that everything should be low-fat or nonfat.

It is important to point out that eating fat does not make you fat. That's right: eating fat is not why you're overweight. To say that eating fat makes you fat sounds catchy and seems to make sense, but it's oversimplifying the issue. Body fat and dietary fat are not the same thing. We need some fat for our bodies to function properly, and there are good fats that we should consume. Not only are they healthy, but they give flavor to food and make us feel full, so we won't overeat.

Fat does have a lot of calories, so eating *a lot* of fat—even healthy fats—will make you gain weight. Eating or drinking more calories than you need from any source, whether it's fat, carbohydrates, or protein, will lead to weight gain. This applies to the AARP New American Diet as well.

I get frustrated, because people try to make healthy choices, but instead they substitute one bad habit for another. I bet it has happened to you. For instance, people follow a diet that is low in fat and instead eat fast carbs: white bread, white rice, potatoes, sugary drinks, and salty snacks. Guess what? Eating too many of these fast carbs is just as bad for your body, and especially your heart and your brain, as eating too much bad fat.

One of my biggest pet peeves is when food manufacturers use the terms *low-fat*, *reduced fat*, or *fat-free*. Many foods you think are healthy actually are not. There are naturally low-fat foods, such as fruits, vegetables, nuts, whole grains, and dried beans; and of course these are healthy choices. But processed foods labeled as low-fat and fat-free are often higher in salt, sugar, or starch than their full-fat counterparts, to make up for the flavor and texture that's lost when the food manufacturers reduce the fat. This makes sense on the surface, since most of us buy food based on taste, and manufacturers want us to buy their food. But they are not necessarily healthy choices.

For example, low-fat and nonfat salad dressings are nearly always higher in sugar and salt. This is very important to know. I've had patients make a great effort to eat more salad, only to become frustrated that they're not losing weight or their cholesterol doesn't improve. Then I find out that they're pouring on salad dressing that has way more calories than the salad!

These fad diets succeed by getting you to reduce your *total number of calories* with no real focus on how the food you are eating affects your *total health.* Yo-yo dieting involves repeatedly losing and regaining body weight. For instance, you lose ten pounds in three months, then regain fifteen pounds in the next two months, then start another diet, and alternate again between losing and gaining weight. This isn't good for your body and has been associated with certain health risks such as high blood pressure and high cholesterol. And as many of you know, it can make it harder to lose weight in the future—both mentally and physically.

Remember the food pyramid? It doesn't exist anymore. It's been replaced by a plate in an attempt to make it simpler. I don't think it is simpler, and I bet you don't, either, although the majority of you probably aren't even familiar with it. It's still too focused on servings, calories, and percentages of nutrients. Healthy eating does not need to be that complicated. And I'm sure many of you don't use a plate to eat all your meals.

The AARP New American Diet doesn't need any gimmicks or tricks to get you to lose weight. It blends the Standard American Diet and the Mediterranean diet into one style of eating that is flavorful, practical, and convenient and that delivers the promise of rapid and sustainable weight loss while reducing the risk of disease. It's solidly based on the NIH-AARP Study. Follow the meal plans for seven, fourteen, or thirty days, and you will see a big difference!

3

AARP New American Diet Nutrition Basics

Knowing what to eat and how your body responds to food is vital as you embark on your journey to weight loss and improved health. This chapter will give you the nutrition basics so you can choose foods that will be not only tasty and nutritious but will also make you healthier.

Deborah Is Tired of Dieting

"Seriously, Dr. Whyte, I'm tired of dieting. I've been doing it for thirty years, and I haven't gotten any thinner. I just can't do it anymore. I drink diet soda—I gain weight. I eat low carbs—I gain weight. I eat high carbs—I gain weight. Nothing works. I've been fat all my life, and that's not going to change. So you might as well save your breath and spare me the food discussion."

That was Deborah's comment after she stepped on the scale. I had not actually said anything yet other than hello.

I responded, "*Diet* is a noun, not a verb. Stop dieting and denying yourself certain food groups or using gimmicks. You need to understand your relationship with food and think of more long-term goals." This is a conversation I've had with Deborah many times.

"I don't even care that much about being overweight," Deborah said. "I'm at that point in my life when I just am tired of feeling tired, and I know my weight isn't helping. I've tried everything, and nothing seems to work."

Deborah had indeed tried numerous fad diets. She tries them for a couple of weeks, and if she doesn't lose any weight, she gives up, thinking she has failed. A few months later she tries another. It's been the same cycle for decades.

"Those fad diets are failing you, Deborah," I told her. "You're not failing them. They don't work long-term."

"I don't know about that, Dr. Whyte. I see them work on some of my friends. My cousin lost twenty pounds on Atkins a few years back," Deborah retorted.

I explained to her that everyone responds to food a little differently. I told her that she needed to focus on the foods for which we have the most information about long-term weight loss, improved health, and even longevity. I reviewed the principles that are in this book: more complex carbohydrates, more whole grains, less processed food, less sugar, less bad fat, more water.

"Dr. Whyte, that's not even a diet, is it?" Deborah asked.

I chuckled. "Actually it is, since I'm using it as a noun!"

"I think I see what you mean," Deborah said with some hesitation. Once I gave her specific meal plans and recipes, she seemed more comfortable with the plan.

I asked her to check in by phone or in person each week for the next four weeks, because I know that Deborah loses interest if she doesn't see immediate results. After the first week, Deborah had lost four pounds.

"That Greek yogurt you recommend is pretty good, and I stay full longer than with the bagel or fruity cereal I had been eating," she commented. I reminded her about the need to closely follow the plan, especially what it includes and excludes.

After two weeks, Deborah had lost an additional four pounds. "I'm starting to see what you mean, Dr. Whyte," she reported. "I don't feel as much as if I'm dieting versus just making smart choices about what to eat."

By the end of the third week, Deborah had lost three more pounds. "I feel like I have more energy nowadays," she said. "I'm not all of a sudden Wonder Woman, but I do think I have a bit more stamina."

At the end of four weeks, Deborah had lost a total of eighteen pounds. "I finally found a diet that actually works for me, and it's not even really a diet," she said excitedly. Before I could say anything, she added, "I'm just joking. I know, I know. It's a different type of diet that forced me to change my way of thinking about food. The best part is that now it just seems natural to eat this way."

Not only do we eat the wrong foods; we also eat much more of them than we should. We have lost all sense of what a normal portion is. Our portion sizes have increased dramatically in the last twenty years. I know many of you often eat out at fast-food restaurants, for both perceived lower cost and convenience. And what do you get at the fast-food joints? The typical meal is a double hamburger or fried chicken, french fries, and, of course, a huge sugar-filled soda. Be honest: How many of you have used the word *supersize* this week?

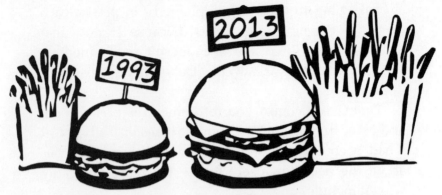

Portion sizes have increased dramatically over the past twenty years,
especially at fast-food restaurants.

I love it when my patients admit that they ate a huge burger
(or two!), supersized fries, and a couple of burritos but then tell
me they had a diet soda—as though the diet soda canceled out all
of those other calories. If only that were true!

AARP New American Diet: The Standard American Diet Meets the Mediterranean Diet

In the Standard American Diet, commonly abbreviated as SAD
(a very appropriate acronym!), we're consuming way too many
calories: close to 3,000 calories daily, when we should be consuming fewer than 2,500 calories per day. We compound the problem
by eating most of those calories in the last third of the day, when
they should be consumed during the first third of the day. As
Americans, we focus on dinner and before-bed snacks and usually
skip breakfast, when we should be starting off the day with a
hearty and healthy meal. And the calories we consume are from
foods filled with saturated fat, trans fat, high levels of sugar, and
refined grains. These are the foods that the NIH-AARP Study has
linked to stroke, heart disease, cancer, and diabetes.

The Mediterranean diet focuses on the eating patterns and
cooking styles of the countries in the Mediterranean region.

The main components are fish, vegetables, fruit, dairy (particularly yogurt and cheese), and moderate wine consumption. Many foods are cooked in olive oil, or it's sprinkled on foods. This type of diet has been shown to reduce heart disease and high blood pressure and may protect the brain from Alzheimer's disease.

How Many Meals a Day Should I Eat?

Part of the Standard American Diet is the idea that we should eat three meals a day: breakfast, lunch, and dinner (although we often don't eat breakfast). But we actually should be eating smaller amounts of food every three to four hours. I'm not suggesting that you eat more food; I'm saying you should eat smaller amounts of food more often. That's also a component of the Mediterranean diet. You'll feel fuller by eating smaller amounts of food more frequently. To understand this, let's go over how your body digests the food you eat.

As soon as we put food into our mouths, our bodies go to work to break it down. Our teeth chew, tearing the food into smaller particles. That's the only part of our digestion we control. Once we start to swallow the food, the body's digestive processes take over and there's nothing we can do about it. You can't consciously tell your colon how to absorb food. (So again, it all starts by you deciding what you put in your mouth.)

The food goes from the mouth to the esophagus and then into the stomach. The stomach is like a churn that mixes the food up, and it also secretes important acids that break down the food particles. Sometimes the acids create problems, such as heartburn or reflux—that's when the acids secreted by the stomach start to dissolve its protective lining or come back up your esophagus.

Several factors affect how long the food stays in our stomach. Carbohydrates spend the least amount of time in the stomach, protein stays in the stomach longer, and fat stays the longest. You'll learn shortly why this is important. As the food particles move into the small intestine, the pancreas and liver get into the act, secreting juices and chemicals that dissolve the food even more. The digested nutrients are absorbed through the intestinal walls and transported throughout the body to help it perform its functions. The remaining particles are pushed into the colon, or large intestine, where they remain until they are expelled by a bowel movement. This entire process is affected by the type and amount of food you eat. Remember, you control this by deciding what you put in your mouth to start the process.

The Role of Insulin

At the simplest level, we eat food for fuel so we can perform physically and mentally in our daily activities. We get the fuel when the body extracts glucose from the foods we eat and converts it into energy. The pancreas is often overlooked in the digestive process, but it plays a very important role when we are trying to lose weight. It secretes the hormone called insulin, which controls the uptake of glucose into your cells.

Insulin is our body's signal to absorb glucose from our blood so our cells can use it as energy. If you have too much glucose in your blood from eating too many foods loaded with sugar and you don't need the glucose for energy right away, the liver converts the excess sugar into glycogen, which is stored in the liver or, more likely, in fat around the body. For some people, all of this excess fat can lead to external obesity, but it also causes a condition in which fat accumulates in and around the liver, which can be quite serious.

When our body needs more energy to perform its functions, it looks for glucose first—either from the food you just ate or from the pancreas, which receives a signal to secrete the hormone glucagon. This converts the glycogen back into glucose, which is then released into your bloodstream for your cells to use. Glucagon is not usually the problem when we're overweight; it's too much sugar, which causes too much insulin release, which causes fat storage.

Our bodies are actually quite good at this process of getting energy from food. They're even better at quickly converting unused glucose into fat—almost too good, since the body doesn't leave unused glucose lying around for very long. It stores it quickly as fat for energy later—energy we usually don't use.

It is important to keep your insulin level low. The AARP New American Diet is going to make sure you manage this critical interaction between glucose and insulin effectively in order to lose weight, refrain from gaining weight, and prevent and manage disease.

• •

What Really Happens When You Eat Those Doughnuts

Let me give you a good example of how this glucose-insulin interaction plays out in your life. As is typical with the Standard American Diet, you probably eat lots of refined carbohydrates for breakfast, such as cornflakes, doughnuts, waffles, various pastries, or bagels. A few minutes later, your digestive system breaks down these high-sugar foods. Lots of sugar in food causes your blood sugar to spike. All of a sudden you have lots of energy, but within an hour your body has released a bunch of insulin, which makes your blood sugar plummet, and now you're sluggish by midmorning. Even worse, you're hungry again!

I know this has happened to you, because it happens to me! That sugar high from the glazed doughnuts doesn't last. Believe me, I've tried it. I feel good for thirty minutes, but within an hour I feel lousy, sleepy, and hungry. So if you tried to improve your diet based on the Standard American Diet, you were set up for failure.

All that sugar in our food is not good. I'm sure you've heard the phrase "garbage in, garbage out." If we're taking in lousy ingredients, we also are going to have lousy energy. Sugar is one of the lousy ingredients we need to cut back on. Did you know that the average sugar consumption for Americans is more than 180 pounds a year per individual? Yes, a year! Some individuals consume more, some consume less. Sugar is the single largest source of calories in the Standard American Diet. You might be thinking, "I only add some sugar to my coffee," but as you'll soon find out, sugar lurks everywhere.

• •

AARP Nutrition Guidelines

What is a calorie? Everyone talks about calories—usually how many you should eat. Calories are important, but I don't think you need to count them.

A calorie is a measure of energy. Technically, one calorie is the amount of energy necessary to raise the temperature of 1 gram of water by 1 degree Celsius. Think of calories as energy you consume as food or energy you expend by being active.

It is often said that "calories in equals calories out." This means that if you put out as much energy (in the form of activity or exercise) as you take in (in the form of calories from food), you'll stay at your current weight. But if you take in more energy than you put out, you'll gain weight. Similarly, if you take in less energy than you put out, you'll lose weight. This is the goal of the AARP New American Diet.

When I first got involved in the issue of obesity as part of the Surgeon General's Call to Action in 2001, I used to think "a calorie is a calorie"—meaning that it doesn't matter where we get our calories from, since the body treats calories the same whether they're from a doughnut, an apple, yogurt, a piece of fish, or a slab of meat.

It turns out that this is not true, and I don't think that way anymore. Where you get your calories from is extremely important, and your choice of the source of calories will determine whether you are overweight. You need to choose calories that are filled with nutrients to improve your health. A large soda may have 250 calories, the same as a piece of fish. Yet even though they have the same calories, the way your body responds to them and the effect they have on your health will be very different.

There are basically two groups of nutrients that you should know about:

- Macronutrients: carbohydrates, fats, protein, and fiber
- Micronutrients: vitamins and minerals

Let's start with the macronutrients.

Carbohydrates

First up: carbohydrates, more commonly known as carbs. I'm sure you've heard of them, but do you know what a carb is or how it might be important to your health?

There are two types of carbs: simple and complex. When you think of a simple carb, think sugar. It can be natural sugar, such as the type found in fruit, or it can be refined sugar, the type typically found in your favorite candy. When you think of a complex carb, think starches, like brown rice and high-fiber foods like oatmeal. It's important to understand the difference between the two types of carbs, because the body responds differently to each.

If a meal has a lot of simple carbs—refined and processed foods, such as a cupcake or a doughnut—you get a burst of energy because your blood sugar spikes. It then drops twenty to thirty minutes later, leaving you feeling sluggish and usually hungry again. Complex carbohydrates provide a slower and more sustained release of energy. That's largely because they take longer to digest—and that's a good thing. This allows glucose to be released into the bloodstream more slowly and more evenly than when we are digesting simple carbs. As we learned in grade school in the story about the tortoise and the hare, "slow and steady wins the race" every time!

Just as there are simple and complex carbs, there are also good and bad carbs. Carbs are an important and useful source of energy for the body. Don't ever let anyone tell you that you don't need carbs; that's wrong. The problem is that we eat too many carbs—and usually the bad ones. Because carbs cause the body to secrete insulin, too many carbs cause too much insulin to be released, which causes too much body fat to be produced and stored. Too much insulin is also a bad thing because it can lead to insulin resistance.

So what do you do? You need to choose the best sources of carbohydrates. I've outlined them in the following lists. You should choose whole grains, fruits, vegetables, and beans. You should avoid the refined, processed carbs, which are quickly digested: white rice, white bread, pastries made from white flour, and sugared sodas. They're the enemy in your weight-loss battle, and you need to eliminate them completely from your diet. If you eat a lot of them now (which you, if you're like most people, probably do), I promise you that the pounds will come off when you get rid of them. I've seen many women who have come down two dress sizes simply by eliminating sugared soda, white rice, and white bread from their diets.

Simple Carbohydrates

Baked goods	Soda
Candy	Sugary breakfast cereals
Fruit	Syrups
Fruit juice	Table sugar
Honey	White bread
Jellies	White pasta
Milk	White rice

Complex Carbohydrates

Beans	Raw vegetables
Brown rice	Seeds
Green vegetables	Sweet potatoes

Lentils	White potatoes
Nuts	Whole-grain bread
Oatmeal	Whole-grain cereals
Onions	Whole-wheat pasta
Peas	

Fats

Fat can be obtained through either animal or vegetable sources in our diet. For most of us, the source is usually animals. If you think about it, we're actually eating an animal's energy reserves—remember, fat is essentially stored energy.

Like carbs, all fats are not created equal. There are two types of fat. They can either be saturated or unsaturated. Let's discuss the bad types first:

- *Saturated fat.* This type of fat is a solid at room temperature. Think *S*: saturated, solid. This type of fat is mostly from animal sources. Common examples are meats and whole-fat dairy products such as whole milk and butter. Saturated fat is also found in coconut and palm oils. Ideally, you should avoid saturated fat because it raises total blood cholesterol and bad, or LDL, cholesterol, both of which increase your risk of heart disease. If you have diabetes, it may be because you eat a lot of saturated fat. We've also learned in the past few years that saturated fat affects sperm count, so men who eat a lot of fatty foods might be reducing their chances of fatherhood.

- *Trans fat.* This type of fat is chemically altered by a process known as *hydrogenation*. The process makes the fat last longer and stay solid, making it easier to cook with and giving the products it's in a longer shelf life. Margarine and vegetable shortening are the most common examples. Highly processed packaged foods often contain trans fat.

Trans fat has been in the news a lot in recent years. It's even more harmful than saturated fat: not only does it increase your total blood cholesterol and bad cholesterol, but it also decreases your good, or HDL, cholesterol. This is exactly the opposite of what you want. We now know that women who eat a lot of trans fat, especially from fried foods and packaged products, are 39 percent more likely to have an ischemic stroke. My advice to you is to avoid trans fat like the plague. You might have to do some detective work when looking at food labels. Manufacturers sometimes say "partially hydrogenated" or "vegetable shortening"—that's trans fat, so if you can avoid it, do so.

The good types of fat are unsaturated, which comes in two kinds:

- *Monounsaturated fat.* This type of fat is found in a variety of plant-based foods and oils, such as olive oil, canola oil, nuts, and avocados. Studies show that a diet (like the Mediterranean diet) that focuses on monounsaturated fats lowers your blood cholesterol levels, which can decrease your risk of heart disease. Research also shows that monounsaturated fats may keep your insulin level low and improve control of your blood sugar, which can be especially helpful if you have type 2 diabetes. That's why this type of fat is good.

- *Polyunsaturated fat.* This type of fat is found mostly in oils, such as sunflower, soybean, cottonseed, or sesame, as well as some nuts, such as walnuts. This is the main type of fat found in fish. Research shows that eating foods rich in polyunsaturated fats lowers the blood cholesterol levels, which can decrease your risk of heart disease. Like monounsaturated fats, polyunsaturated fats may also decrease the risk of type 2 diabetes.

You probably have heard about polyunsaturated fat because a particular type is omega-3 fatty acids. Omega-3, found in some types of fatty fish (such as salmon), reduces your chances of getting a heart attack. It also prevents irregular heartbeat, lowers blood pressure levels, reduces joint pain, and even builds brain cell membranes. In fact, a recent study showed that people with low levels of omega-3 fatty acids had brains with less volume compared to the brains of people who had higher levels of omega-3. This may translate to faster aging of the brain and worse cognitive function. The NIH-AARP Study has shown that omega-3 fatty acids might also play a role in preventing cancer and some inflammatory conditions such as rheumatoid arthritis. Pretty powerful stuff!

I probably should spend a little more time here discussing omega-3 fatty acids, because most people don't know that our bodies cannot make them; we get them only through food or supplements. That's why what we choose to eat is so important and so powerful. There are two major types of omega-3 fatty acids: (1) alpha-linolenic acid (ALA), found in some vegetable oils, such as soybean, canola, and flaxseed oils; in walnuts; and in some green vegetables, such as brussels sprouts, kale, spinach, and salad greens; and (2) eicosapentaenoic acid (EPA) and docosa-hexaenoic acid (DHA); EPA and DHA are the types of omega-3 found in fatty fish.

This is one reason fish is so important. I will be emphasizing fish as part of your new diet because it's the major source of omega-3 fatty acids, a nutrient that we need to be eating more of. We simply do not get enough.

There are also omega-6 fatty acids (linoleic acid). You might not have heard of them. These are found mostly in vegetable oils like soybean, corn, and safflower oils. Omega-6 fatty acids lower bad cholesterol and reduce inflammation. Unlike omega-3, however, omega-6 tends to be prevalent in our diet, so I typically don't worry about getting enough omega-6, and you shouldn't, either. Both omega-6 and omega-3 fatty acids are healthy. I mention this because some of you who follow diet information might have heard a theory in the past that omega-3 fatty acids are better for our health than omega-6 fatty acids, but that is not supported by the latest evidence.

• •

Is It Better to Get Omega-3 Fatty Acids from Food or from Supplements?

Ideally, you should get omega-3 fatty acids from food, since the foods that contain them have other vital nutrients your body can use. I always recommend eating foods rather than popping supplements. If you don't like fish, however, I do recommend that you take an omega-3 supplement daily. The American Heart Association recommends one gram per day of fish oil containing EPA and DHA for those with documented coronary heart disease, preferably from oily fish, although supplements are okay with a doctor's approval. For those without documented heart disease, the AHA recommends just eating a variety of fish, preferably oily, twice a week. Don't increase that dosage without consulting your doctor, since more than 3 grams can cause bleeding.

Some recent studies suggest that if you have heart disease, you might benefit from two doses a day. But check with your doctor. There is a type of omega-3 fatty acid pill available by prescription that can help if you have very high triglycerides.

• •

Good Fats

Monounsaturated:
  Almonds
  Avocados
  Canola oil
  Cashews
  Hazelnuts
  Macadamia nuts
  Olive oil
  Olives
  Peanut butter

    Peanuts
    Pistachios
    Sesame oil
    Sunflower oil
    Sunflower seeds
Polyunsaturated:
    Brazil nuts
    Chia seeds
    Fatty fish (tuna, trout, salmon, mackerel)
    Pecans
    Pine nuts
    Pumpkin seeds
    Safflower oil
    Sesame seeds
    Soybean oil
    Tofu
    Walnuts

Bad Fats
Saturated:
    Cocoa butter
    Coconut oil
    Palm oil
    Poultry
    Red meat
    Whole-fat dairy
Trans:
    Cake and cookie mixes
    Candy bars
    Commercially baked goods
    Crackers
    Fried foods
    Frozen dinners
    Margarine
    Microwave popcorn
    Packaged snack goods (potato chips, for example)

Protein

Protein has been in the news quite a bit in the past few years, given that various fad diets have focused on protein. Let me give you some background.

Our bodies use protein for a variety of functions, including cell growth and repair. Protein is also necessary to make antibodies to fight infections, and it even keeps our bones strong. So having protein as part of your diet is pretty important to keep you healthy. Some nutritionists even suggest we consume 1 gram of protein per day for every 2 pounds of normal body weight.

A protein is basically a chain of amino acids. There are some amino acids that we need to survive and that our body cannot make, so we have to consume them as part of our diet. They are called *essential amino acids*. Just like carbs and fat, proteins may be divided into two types: complete and incomplete. A *complete* protein source provides all of the eight essential amino acids. You may also hear these sources called *high-quality proteins*. These are typically animal-based foods, such as red meat, poultry, fish, milk, yogurt, eggs, and cheese. An *incomplete* protein source is low in one or more of the essential amino acids. Examples are grains, nuts, seeds, beans, and peas. These can be combined with one another to make a complete protein (for example, beans and rice).

Because of the complicated biochemical structure of proteins, they can be hard to digest. The body actually has to work to digest them and puts out energy to consume them. As a result, they are absorbed slowly during the digestive process. But slow is good when we're talking about digestion.

The Power of Fiber

Fiber is technically a type of carbohydrate. But for our purposes, it's different, since it is not digested. So I want to talk about it separately. It's often underemphasized in any type of weight-loss strategy, and that's a mistake. I don't want you to overlook the power of fiber.

Fiber resists digestive enzymes and cannot be absorbed by your body. Just like everything else I've been discussing, fiber has two types: soluble and insoluble.

Soluble fiber dissolves in water. This type of fiber is found in apples, pears, strawberries, blueberries, oats, and barley as well as in beans, peas, lentils, and nuts. Soluble fiber lowers cholesterol. It's also important because it slows the uptake of glucose, which helps to maintain a healthy blood sugar level. This can help prevent diabetes.

Insoluble fiber doesn't dissolve in water. Our parents usually called it "roughage." This type of fiber is found in whole grains (such as brown rice), seeds, carrots, cucumbers, zucchini, celery, dark leafy vegetables, onions, raisins, grapes, and tomatoes. This type of fiber promotes bowel health—basically, it keeps you regular. It does this by regulating the speed at which food moves through the intestines; adjusting the speed prevents you from getting constipated. This type of fiber bulks up your stool and makes it softer by absorbing water.

Another great thing about fiber is that it tends to make you feel full longer and can curb overeating. Sometimes people don't like high-fiber foods because they can require a lot more chewing than we're used to—but that can be a good thing. Taking longer to chew will prevent you from putting too much food in your mouth. As with everything else, however, you can get too much of a good thing. Too much fiber, as you may know, can lead to gas or diarrhea and in some rare cases, even obstruction.

Vitamins and Minerals

Vitamins and minerals have no calories yet are still critical for obtaining and maintaining good health.

Vitamins are organic nutrients that enable our bodies to use the macronutrients. Vitamins fall into two categories: fat-soluble and water-soluble. The fat-soluble vitamins—A, D, E, and K—dissolve in fat and can be stored in your body. The water-soluble vitamins—C and B-complex (such as folate and niacin)—need to dissolve in water before your body can absorb them. As a result, your body can't store these vitamins. Any vitamin C or B that your body doesn't use is typically eliminated by the end of the day through your urine. So you need a fresh supply of these water-soluble vitamins daily. That's the major difference between the two types of vitamins, and this is why what you put into your body every day is so important.

I know my young nephews think of certain types of stones and rocks when I mention minerals, and in some ways they are right. Whereas vitamins are organic substances made by plants or animals, minerals are inorganic elements that come from the soil, rocks, and water. Our bodies need minerals to perform many functions, such as strengthening bones and maintaining a normal heart rate. The classic mineral that nutritionists like to talk about is calcium, a very important mineral for good health. It seems kind of strange to say your body also needs minerals such as copper, iron, magnesium, sulfur, iodine, chromium, and zinc, but you do! Remember, you are eating only very small amounts of these as part of a healthy diet.

The best way to get enough vitamins and minerals is to eat a variety of foods that includes carbohydrates, fat, and protein. You don't want to completely exclude any of the macronutrients as part of a plan to lose weight and live longer.

• •

Should I Take a Multivitamin?

Vitamins are an important component of a healthy eating plan. I find that patients are often interested in consuming multivitamins, as though they have magical effects. Do you remember when vitamin C was the rage years ago, and we thought it was going to be a cure for every malady? Some of my patients still do.

No one particular component of a healthy eating plan outweighs all of the other components. Consuming too few vitamins can cause problems, but so can consuming too many. The truth is that most of us get enough vitamins A, C, and E through our diet, even if we don't eat as healthily as we should. Since the AARP New American Diet is teaching you about healthy eating, there's no need for you to take a multivitamin. And the NIH-AARP Study found that for men, overuse of multivitamins can put them at increased risk of prostate cancer.

The one vitamin I do talk about to patients is vitamin D, which has been in the news in recent years. If you don't get enough vitamin D, you can develop weak bones as well as increase your risk for stroke and dementia. As we age, our skin loses the ability to make the precursor of vitamin D. The Institute of Medicine recommends 600 international units (IU) for adults ages fifty to seventy years old and 800 IU for adults older than seventy. Your skin color, your age, the amount of time you spend in the sun, and where you live affect the amount of vitamin D your body makes. Instead of automatically supplementing patients with vitamin D, I check their levels, and that way I know for sure. If their levels are low, I will either review their diets or recommend supplementation. As with everything else, you can get too much of a good thing, and too much vitamin D can actually erase the benefit it has for the heart.

• •

Dietary Sources of Vitamins

Vitamin A: carrots, kale, collard greens, orange fruits (cantaloupe, apricots, peaches, mangoes), spinach, sweet potatoes, chicken liver.

Vitamin B: eggs, tuna, salmon, turkey, beans, lentils, chard, chicken, beef, whole wheat, spinach, nuts, bananas.

Vitamin C: grapefruit, tomatoes, oranges, broccoli, brussels sprouts, kale, kiwi, strawberries, red and green peppers.

Vitamin D: salmon, cheese, eggs, mushrooms, milk, flounder, pork, tuna, ricotta cheese.

Vitamin E: eggs, sunflower seeds, almonds, spinach, olives, turnip greens, whole grains, hazelnuts.

In This Diet, There's No Calorie Counting!

Studies have consistently shown that if you eat too many calories (consume more calories through food than you put out through activity or exercise), you will gain weight. It doesn't matter if the calories are from carbohydrates, fat, or protein. Calories count, but you don't need to count calories. It's not practical or realistic, and it's often hard to get accurate information.

One of my first projects when I started working at the Discovery Channel was to create a video in which we went to a food court and asked people to estimate the number of calories in their meals. (You can view it at www.health.discovery.com /videos/health-vignettes-hidden-calories-in-the-food-court .html.) Guess what? People consistently underestimated the number of calories by a third. And scientific studies have also demonstrated this at least a dozen times. A recent study showed that only 9 percent of us can accurately estimate the number of calories in a meal. Most people just aren't good at doing it, and even when the number of calories is listed on a label, it is not always accurate.

We also aren't good at estimating the number of calories we burn. Studies have shown that people vastly overestimate the number of calories they burn while walking or exercising. I have a group of patients who are part of a walking club. They walk a couple of miles in the morning about three days a week. When they are done with their morning hike, they go to the local pancake shop to celebrate the fact that they got up early and walked. I asked some of them once how many calories they think they burned; they responded by saying 1,000 calories, when the true number was probably around 300 calories—almost the amount of one large soda. They were under the false impression that since they were burning a lot of calories through walking, they could eat more.

I was happy that they understood the concept of "calories in equals calories out" and how that leads to weight maintenance. The problem was that they were using inaccurate numbers on both sides of the equation. The counters on the exercise equipment at the gym that supposedly tell you how many calories you are burning are notoriously inaccurate—those machines can't possibly tell how hard you are working. So all this counting is just too complicated and fraught with error.

More important, the goal of losing weight is to live a healthier life, feel better, become pain-free, and be more vital—not just to see a lower number on the scale by counting calories. Counting calories misses the big picture. What you put in your mouth is as important as what you don't put in; what you include in your meals is as important as what you exclude. With the knowledge you gain from this book, you'll automatically choose foods that are filled with healthy nutrients and eat them in the right amounts and at the right times. It'll become natural for you to make the healthy choice instead of the unhealthy choice. And you won't even need to think about it after a while—it'll become automatic. No calculators are required.

4

You Don't Have to Be Overweight

Let's start with definitions. What does it mean to be overweight? You step on a scale and it gives you a number, but how do you know how to interpret it? It's just a number, isn't it? *Overweight* is defined as an excessively high amount of body fat in relation to lean body mass. Scientifically, *overweight* refers to increased body weight in relation to height, which is then compared to a standard of acceptable weight. Body mass index (BMI) is the common measure we use to express the relationship of weight to height.

It's important that you know your BMI, because that lets you know if you are of normal weight, overweight, or obese. You cannot look at yourself in the mirror, pinch your belly, and decide whether you need to lose a few pounds. I know many of you do that, but it doesn't work. I still remember the "pinch an inch" commercials for a certain type of cereal, and I too would often pinch my stomach to determine if I needed to lose weight. Today we need a little more information to determine a healthy weight than just how much flesh we feel when we pinch ourselves.

The equation is pretty simple:

$$BMI = \frac{weight\ (lb) * 703}{height^2\ (in^2)}$$

OR

$$BMI = \frac{weight\ (kg)}{height^2\ (m^2)}(metric)$$

You don't even need to do the math yourself. You can easily calculate it online at www.nhlbisupport.com/bmi or aarp.org/healthtools. All you need to know is your weight and your height (which you need to measure only once, but please have someone else measure it—some people, especially men, say they are taller than they actually are).

Once you know your BMI, you can determine whether you need to lose weight and, if so, how much you need to lose.

What BMI Numbers Indicate

17.5–18.5: Underweight
18.5–24.9: Normal weight
25–29.9: Overweight
30–40: Obese
>40: Morbidly obese

Most people really don't know how much they weigh or how much they should weigh. That's why the information I'm giving you is both easy and important. For example, if you're five feet five and weigh 156 pounds, your BMI is 26, which puts you in the category of overweight. Following the chart, you should weigh between 114 and 144 pounds. If you're four feet eleven and weigh 148 pounds, you have a BMI of 30, which is considered obese. You need to weigh between 94 and 119 pounds.

So how much do you weigh? What's your BMI? How much should you weigh? It's a good idea to record these figures here since we'll come back to this when we talk about goals.

Date:
My weight:
My BMI:
My healthy weight range:
Number of pounds I need to lose:

But I'm Not Fat—I'm Muscular!

BMI has come under some controversy in the past few years because it does not take into account how muscular a person is. Therefore, the definitions of overweight and obesity as determined by BMI do not apply to a very fit athlete or muscular person. That's partly because muscle weighs more than fat, so a muscular person's excess weight is not necessarily harmful.

But let's be realistic—99 percent of us are not in that category. A few middle-age men have said to me, "Dr. Whyte, I'm not overweight; I'm muscular." Honestly, that has never been the case; they've never been so muscular that it skewed the definition for them. For most of us, if our BMI is high, it's not because we have too much muscle. So let's stop kidding ourselves.

The Size of Your Waist

Waist circumference is another important measure. By this, I mean the fat around the belly. Belly fat is especially concerning, because it releases harmful substances such as adipokines, which raise our blood pressure; mess up our blood sugar, causing diabetes; and even put us at risk of having a heart attack. The information I present in this book will help you get rid of the fat in your belly—and you need to get rid of it if you want to be healthy.

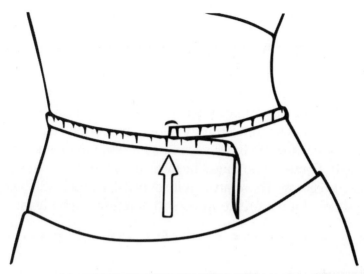

To measure your waist circumference, place a tape measure around your waist, level with your belly button. Make sure that the tape measure is not too tight and that it is parallel to the floor.

How do you measure the size of your waist? It's not the waist size of your pants or skinny jeans or your belt size. There's little correlation between your pants size and the true size of your waist. How many of you squeeze yourselves into your pants? (I know, I know, the dryer shrank them!) To measure your waist circumference, take a tape measure, start at the top of the hip bone, and bring the tape measure all the way around—level it with your belly button. Make sure it's not too tight and that it is parallel to the floor. Do not suck in your gut or hold your breath while doing it. We want accurate information.

Waist Circumference

Men: should be less than 40 inches
Women: should be less than 35 inches

Keep in mind that this information is useful only for people with a BMI between 25.5 and 34.9. It is not useful if you have a BMI over 35, since you are already at an increased risk.

• •

DXA: A Test to Measure Body Fat

If you really want to know for sure how much body fat you have, there may be a new test on the horizon. The most accurate test to measure body fat is a special scan called DXA, which stands for dual-energy X-ray absorptiometry. It precisely measures body fat as well as muscle mass and bone density. Some of you might be familiar with it from osteoporosis screening. This scan is quite expensive and is still being used only for research purposes in determining body fat.

• •

Now it's your turn:
My waist circumference:

How Often Should You Weigh Yourself?

You're probably wondering how often you should weigh yourself. Weighing yourself is an important step in losing weight. Without the information about your weight, you can never know for sure how serious an issue your weight is or how well you are doing once you start your weight-loss plan.

I've learned in the last twenty years that people consistently underestimate their weight. I used to joke that I wished patients weighed only as much as they thought they did. At least once a week someone would say, "Gosh, I didn't realize I gained that much weight." Studies have shown that overweight and obese women often have wrong perceptions of their bodies and how much they weigh. Among obese women, approximately 80 percent underestimate their weight. Nearly 50 percent of overweight women do, compared with 13 percent of normal-weight women. This goes back to my "Stop kidding yourself" mantra. You know you've gained weight; knowing how much is an important step in reversing it.

When you're doing well and losing weight, the information can be a great motivator to keep up the good work. When you're not losing weight, however, knowing the information can make you lose all motivation. I've seen it many times personally and professionally. It's human nature.

We'll talk more later about how to reprogram your brain about your weight, but you should know this: numerous studies have shown that men and women who weigh themselves weekly during a weight-loss regimen lose more weight than those who don't.

Weigh yourself once a week, but no more, for the first month, and then every other week for the second and third months. Keep a chart of your weight to keep track of it.

Weight Fluctuation

Your weight can fluctuate as much as four or five pounds throughout the course of the day. It's normal and is the result of a number of factors—mostly how your body handles water through processes such as sweating and urinating. Water actually weighs quite a bit, so if you weigh yourself after drinking a lot of water, the scale number might be a little higher than you expected. Don't worry, though, because water is quickly eliminated from your body. Don't avoid water in an attempt to drop pounds, since not drinking enough water can actually also cause the scale number to increase. This happens because if you don't drink enough water, the body will attempt to retain water, and it's usually successful in doing so. That's why drinking water can actually help you to lose weight long-term. You'll read more about that in the upcoming chapters.

I often suggest to people that they weigh themselves at the same time of day, either first thing in the morning, after you empty your bladder and before you take a shower, or at night, right before you go to bed. And believe it or not, clothes really don't weigh that much, so if you don't want to weigh yourself in your underwear, that's okay.

Weight, Sex, and Race

In general, more women than men are overweight. Twice as many women as men are morbidly obese. There are several reasons for this.

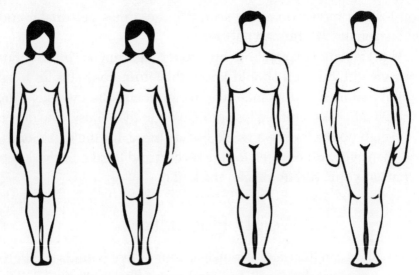

Women and men who are of normal weight and overweight.

Men tend to be shaped like apples, whereas women tend to be shaped like pears. Men build up fat in the stomach area; women store their fat around the hips, buttocks, and thighs. The reasons for this date back centuries, and we're not going to change it. Women store fat in those areas to help with pregnancy and breast-feeding.

In addition, up until our fifties, men have less body fat than women, primarily because men have about 20 percent more skeletal muscle mass. That affects their shape. Men get an added benefit, because muscle burns more calories than fat does; so even when they're just sitting there doing nothing, men burn more calories than women. I know it's not fair, but that's just how we have evolved.

Adult obesity rates for blacks and Hispanics are considerably higher than for whites. The obesity rate in whites is 34 percent, in Hispanics it is 39 percent, and in African Americans it is 49 percent. What's truly shocking is that over half of all African American women and over 40 percent of Mexican American women are obese. As a result, African American and Hispanic women suffer from higher rates of diabetes, heart disease, cancer, high blood pressure, arthritis, and other serious health problems than the rest of the population does.

Weight and Age

I'm sure many of you have noticed that as you are getting older, you are putting on more weight and your body shape seems to be changing. We gain about ten pounds each decade, starting in our twenties, and it continues to our mid-fifties. For many of us, that can add up to forty to fifty pounds. Most of it is fat, and that's another reason our body shape changes. One pound of fat takes up nearly 20 percent more space than a pound of muscle mass does, so the extra fat makes us larger—literally. At the same time, starting in our mid-twenties, we begin to lose muscle mass if we don't do anything about it. Unfortunately, that's exactly when many people stop going to the gym or being active. The result is that we lose about a quarter pound of muscle every year from ages twenty-five to fifty and then a pound of muscle every year from our fifties on. This may not sound like much, but over twenty or thirty years it really adds up.

• •

Menopause and Weight Gain

Weight gain and changes in fat distribution typically occur after menopause. It's mainly because there is a decline in estrogen and progesterone. These hormones affect the fat cells in a way that causes more fat to be deposited centrally in our bodies. Hormonal changes also cause a woman's body to retain more water all over, causing weight gain.

By menopause, two-thirds of women have become overweight. Estrogen replacement therapy does not prevent the weight gain, although it may minimize fat redistribution. Estrogen replacement does have some risks, and it is not recommended as part of a weight-loss plan.

• •

"But My Genes Make Me Fat!"

Many patients have told me that there is nothing they can do about their weight, because, they say, "I was born fat!" At least once a month, a patient declares to me, "Dr. Whyte, I have the fat gene."

What exactly is the role of genetics? Some data show that obesity starts in the womb—but not in the way you might think. Women who are significantly overweight when they become pregnant often have babies who are nearly obese by the time they are nine months old. Most research shows that it's because of the quantity of food the new moms feed their newborns. After all, we are not programmed to become overweight—or are we?

Some people believe in a *set point* for weight—the belief that we are programmed genetically to weigh a certain number of pounds, and our bodies will work to achieve that weight. This theory presumes that everyone has a different set point. My set point might be 170 pounds, whereas yours might be 150 pounds. In an underfed state, with the resulting weight loss, the body will reduce its energy expenditure, which reduces the rate of weight loss. In an overfed state, the body will rev up the metabolism to burn calories, restoring you to the body's biological set point.

This theory has never been proved, and most doctors and scientists discount it. I mention it because some patients still mention it, thinking that somehow they are programmed to be overweight, but that simply isn't the case. To make matters worse, if you believe you are destined to be fat, you are less likely to change your behavior. After all, why bother? A recent study showed that when overweight patients were told they had "fat-promoting genes," they were more likely to eat fatty foods because they thought being fat was their genetic fate and there was nothing they could do about it. They truly are mistaken.

When we talk about genes, we need to understand that changes in the gene pool occur over hundreds, if not thousands, of years. The obesity epidemic is a relatively new phenomenon, of the past thirty to forty years. So despite what some of you may think, your genes are not making you fat. Even if there is a role for genetics, it would only make you predisposed to gain weight, but the environment—what you eat, how much you eat, and how much you exercise—plays a more important role.

Your Weight, Your Life Span

So why does all this matter? As I mentioned earlier, weight and life span are connected. The harsh reality is that the risk of early death rises with an increasing BMI, and that risk increases dramatically with a BMI greater than 30. If your BMI is over 30, your risk of early death is two or three times higher than it is for people who have a BMI of 20 to 25. You are doubling and tripling your risk of early death by being overweight. Obesity causes diseases that kill more than 110,000 Americans a year. That's why this book, which is largely based on the NIH-AARP Study, is so important.

Please don't shorten your life span by eating the wrong foods. Being overweight increases your chances of developing serious health conditions that include high blood pressure, high cholesterol, diabetes, heart disease, stroke, arthritis, gallstones, incontinence, sleep apnea, and cancer. Some of you may already have some of these conditions.

I know many of you are concerned about Alzheimer's. Did you know that the risk of developing dementia increases 3.6 times if you have a high BMI? (So if you're doing Sudoku to help with brain function, you might want to do it while you're on the treadmill!)

Preliminary studies suggest that overeating may double your risk of memory loss. Scientists recently discovered that older people who ate more than 2,100 calories a day had more than double the rate of memory loss called mild cognitive impairment. The more calories consumed, the more likely people were to develop memory loss.

I've seen the diagnosis of sleep apnea increase dramatically in the past few years, and it's directly related to excess weight. Think of it this way: being overweight has almost as many health risks as smoking, and we all know that smoking is bad for you. As the

NIH-AARP Study confirmed, the longer you are overweight or obese, the more problems you are going to develop. Your excess weight causes many of your health problems, and deep down I think you know that.

Can You Be Overweight and Still Be Fit?

Being fit might actually trump being fat, according to some researchers. But what is considered *fit*? If you are fit like a Navy SEAL, you can do forty-two push-ups in two minutes, fifty-two sit-ups in two minutes, and eight pull-ups followed by a one-and-a-half-mile run within eleven and a half minutes.

For your purpose, however, you could be considered fit and overweight if you can walk thirty to sixty minutes without having to stop, climb two flights of stairs without becoming winded, and do moderate aerobic activity such as a short jog. In addition, you would need to be physically active five hours a week to meet the criteria of *fit*. If you meet this definition, you reduce your risk of developing health problems from your excess weight. It doesn't mean you eliminate risk, you simply reduce it.

Before you go out and put on your running shoes, you should know that diet is roughly 70 percent of the work for losing weight or maintaining a healthy weight; exercise is certainly important, but it represents only 30 percent of the work. And if you're looking for those elusive abs, you can do two hundred crunches a day, but unless you lose the body fat, the six-pack will never appear.

• •

Medicare and Obesity

If you're a Medicare beneficiary, Medicare will pay for obesity counseling. Beneficiaries with BMI values of 30 or more can receive weekly in-person intensive behavioral therapy visits for one month, followed by visits every two weeks for an additional five months, fully paid for by Medicare with no copayment. Additional monthly sessions will be covered for up to another six months if the beneficiary has lost at least 6.6 pounds during the first six months. More details can be found at www.cms.gov.

• •

Avoid Diet Soda!

One of the best examples of having to cut through the clutter is the issue of diet soda. Believe it or not, diet soda might actually cause you to *gain* weight. How is this possible? After all, shouldn't these zero-calorie beverages help you achieve your weight-loss goal? Aren't they "free" calories? The drinks may be free of calories, but they are not free of consequences. It turns out that we need to look at the effect of sugar substitutes on the brain. When we eat, signals from the tongue tell the brain that food is on the way, and the brain coordinates the rest of the body to expect a flood of calories.

Sugar substitutes in diet soda, like aspartame, sucralose, and saccharin, are so chemically similar to sugar that they fool our taste buds and brains into thinking that we are eating real sugar. Remember those soda taste-test commercials from years ago? Consumers couldn't tell the difference between diet and regular soda. Well, these people were not acting—their brains really couldn't tell the difference!

Once the brain gets the body ready for calories, our desire to eat is activated and gets ramped up until those calories are received. Instead of diet soda squelching our appetites, it may instead motivate us to eat, and this, of course, can easily thwart the golden rule of dieting: fewer calories in than out. Add to this the fact that sweetness as a taste can have addictive properties, and suddenly sugar substitutes, which to the brain "taste" many more times as sweet as regular sugar, might increase the craving to get those calories from the sweets that you're working so hard to keep out. Ugh!

Some researchers also believe that people drinking diet soda overestimate the number of calories they are saving, and this results in overeating, and then weight gain. We all have ordered those big meals and then drunk a diet soda hoping it all balances out—but it doesn't.

Hormones Can Sabotage Weight Loss

Our bodies and our hormones can actually sabotage our efforts to lose weight and keep it off. A recent study examined overweight adults who lost thirty pounds by reducing the number of calories they consumed. For ten weeks, the researchers measured the levels of various hormones before and after they lost the weight.

Guess what? A hormone known as leptin, which is associated with feeling full and satisfied, dropped significantly after the weight loss and stayed low for a year. That's a bad thing, because when leptin is released it decreases our appetite and increases our body's ability to burn fat. We want more leptin around when we're trying to lose weight.

The same is true for a hormone called peptide YY, which suppresses hunger; in people who have been losing weight over time, peptide YY becomes abnormally low. And ghrelin, a hormone that increases hunger, actually rose and remained high for up to a year in the study. Again, a bad thing. Ghrelin should be lower, not higher, if we want to lose weight. This explains why it's so hard to keep the weight off.

The body experiences weight loss as a stress and kicks into high gear to fight the stressor. Along with changing the hormone levels to hold on to the remaining weight and even regain lost weight, the body slows down its basal metabolic rate to maintain pounds. Our bodies aren't trying to do the wrong thing on purpose; that's just how some of us have our brains and our bodies wired.

Soon you will learn ways you can rewire the neurocircuitry so you don't regain weight, and thereby reach and maintain a healthy weight through eating foods that directly improve your health. Losing weight is as much about the brain as it is about the body. I often tell patients that the key to weight loss is right between your ears. It's your brain, not your mouth.

Nancy's Diabetes Story

Nancy is a forty-four-year-old woman who has had diabetes for three years. When I started working with her, her BMI was 28, on the high side. "I've always been a bit heavy" was her usual refrain, and she was pretty resistant to change. She had an excuse for every suggestion I made. "I don't like the taste of water." "I don't like the smell of fish." "Salads don't fill me up enough." She was taking metformin for diabetes and a blood pressure medication for high blood pressure. Her blood sugars were poorly controlled.

Nancy had been gaining weight steadily over the past few years, and if her blood sugar didn't improve, insulin injections would be the next step. "Dr. Whyte, I am not going to use needles," she told me. "They make me faint." I explained that insulin is actually a very good drug and might prevent complications from diabetes that are likely to occur in a few years if we don't control her blood sugar.

"I'll do anything to avoid the needle," she said. Given this new motivation, we discussed a weight-loss plan that focused on whole grains, fish, water, and nuts. It also included a graduated exercise program.

At her one-month visit, she had lost eight pounds, and her blood sugars were slightly improved. "I didn't realize all the different types of fish out there," she told me.

At her two-month visit, Nancy had lost another four pounds, and her blood sugars were almost in the normal range. "I actually feel healthier, Dr. Whyte," she told me, "and I no longer am eating any sweets. I bet you didn't

realize I had been secretly eating sweets all these years."
I smiled.

By her three-month visit, she had lost an additional six pounds. She had now lost more than 10 percent of her previous body weight. Not only did she not need to start insulin, I actually took her off the metformin because her blood sugars were markedly improved. I even lowered her blood pressure medication since her blood pressure readings were improved.

"Although you told me about it," Nancy said, "I really didn't make the connection between food and how it affected my diabetes until I actually saw it with my own eyes. Now I believe it, and I'm more careful about what I eat."

5

Dealing with Emotional Eating and Cravings

Susan and Snacking

Susan is a fifty-one-year-old woman who has struggled with weight issues most of her adult life. "Up until college, Dr. Whyte, I used to be as thin as a pencil," she told me. "But in college, I developed bad eating habits and have been trying to break them ever since."

Susan is about five feet four; when she came to me a few months ago, she weighed nearly 160 pounds, so she had a bit of weight to lose. At the visit, she declared she was going to lose weight. "Just like you've said, I need to eat more often. So I'm going to start snacking," she said.

"That's great, Susan. I have some suggestions about what to eat," I replied.

"It can't be that complicated, Dr. Whyte," she responded. "I'll call you if I have any questions."

A month later, I got a call from Susan. "I might need your help on this snacking. I haven't lost any weight. I've actually gained two pounds," she remarked.

"What have you been snacking on?" I asked.

"I bought these granola bars that I eat every day in between breakfast and lunch," she said. "Then I've been eating some low-fat crackers and drinking diet soda around three o'clock. But I'll be honest; sometimes candy looks pretty appetizing after the crackers and soda."

I gently pointed out the problems with these choices. Granola bars are notorious for having lots of sugar and unhealthy oils. "Is it chewy?" I asked her what brand of bar she was eating, since some are healthier than others.

"Yes, it's better than those hard dry ones," Susan said. I pointed out to her that it's usually molasses that makes it chewy. Often the chewier it is, the less healthy it is. As for the diet soda, I explained to her that the artificial sweetener is tricking her brain into getting her body ready for something sweet. When she doesn't get it, it makes her crave it even more. "I thought it seemed odd that I felt like eating a cupcake with the diet soda. I thought I was just going crazy!" Susan exclaimed.

I suggested that she just drink water. I also recommended nuts as a snack, as well as string cheese and whole-wheat crackers. And I advised her that fruit is a great way to satisfy that sweet tooth of hers.

Two weeks later, Susan called me and said, "You had some good suggestions, Dr. Whyte. It took a few days to get used to what you suggested, but it really seems to work. The nuts especially fill me up, and I even feel healthier drinking lots of water. I bring an apple to work most days, and now even my kids are eating fruit. I've only lost five pounds so far, but this smart snacking is something I'm going to do no matter what."

Why We Eat

Many patients have said to me, "Dr. Whyte, the problem is that sometimes I don't even know why I eat." I bet you have felt that way at times. It's the classic "I'm not even hungry, but I'm eating anyway."

Our brains have a tremendous effect on how, when, and why we eat. Some of us eat when we are depressed, and some of us don't eat when we are stressed or anxious. Most of us eat to celebrate successes and special occasions such as birthdays, anniversaries, or job promotions. And, of course, we celebrate by eating when we lose a lot of weight in time for a special event. You know what I'm talking about. Many of us eat when we aren't even hungry, or we eat when we think we are hungry, but we really are not, in the true sense of the word.

I promised that I would give you more power, and now is the time for you to learn how to use your brain to eat healthily, have more vitality, think more clearly, lose weight, and reduce your risk of disease.

I'll be honest—I wasn't always a big believer in the mind-body connection. As I've matured and learned more medicine and have become friends with physicians who take an integrative medical approach, including Drs. Mehmet Oz and Dean Ornish, I've become a firm believer that our minds can affect our health tremendously, and this includes how much we weigh. Never underestimate the power of your mind to change your body!

Why Do You Want to Lose Weight?

One of the first things I talk about with patients when we discuss weight-loss strategies is why they want to lose weight. Not everyone has the same motivation. What is yours? Do you think that if you lose weight, you will look more attractive? Do you want to have more energy, more vitality, and less joint pain? Or do you know that all of those excess pounds might eventually make you sick and die sooner than you should? There's no right answer, but to achieve success, you need to have a reason to change. When you face the ups and downs of weight loss, the underlying reason you want to lose weight will help you to prevail through the rough times and the false starts.

You need a long-term reason, not just that you want to look sexy for an upcoming reunion. You need to be in this to feel better for life and to make sure your life doesn't end prematurely because of what you choose to feed yourself.

Emotional Eating

To be successful with any plan to lose weight, you need to understand and examine your relationship with food. I bet some of you reading this feel powerless when it comes to food. But you don't have to be.

Take a few minutes to reflect on how you think of food. Some of us are emotional eaters. We eat food—typically high-fat, sugary food such as ice cream—that makes us feel good. Eating that kind of food seems to elevate our mood and relieve our stress a little. And the food might actually do that, as you'll soon find out. Does that describe you?

Others eat partly because it's hard to sit still. We need to be doing something, especially with our hands. So eating keeps us busy. Does that describe you?

Then there are other folks—normal-weight and skinny people—who don't eat at all when they are upset or anxious. My mother is like that; whenever she is upset over something, she doesn't want to eat anything. Other people when stressed prefer to eat, eat, and eat. Knowing your relationship with food will help you to understand why you eat certain foods, and this knowledge will give you the power to change your behavior.

Fundamentally, you should be eating food when you are truly hungry, not because you're stressed, bored, lonely, tired, or unhappy. You probably eat sometimes not because you are hungry but because, in your mind, it's time to eat. You might eat because it has become a habit. People have told me they drink a soda every day at three o'clock because it's become a routine—not because they are thirsty. Others tell me they eat ice cream every night while they watch their favorite television show because that's what they're used to doing. They're not eating because they need sustenance; they may convince themselves they're hungry, but they're really not.

I sometimes recommend to certain patients that they eat nothing for ten hours—absolutely nothing. That way, they can actually remember what it feels like to be truly hungry.

If you want to lose weight and keep it off, understanding your relationship with food is a key to success. Weight loss is not going to be achieved through studying food labels and counting calories, but rather by you gaining more self-respect and valuing yourself. When you begin to understand your relationship with food and care about how you look and feel, you'll begin to make healthy choices.

Food Can Be Like a Drug

It also helps to understand how the brain reacts to food and how that affects the body. Remember when I said that food is like a drug? Just as drugs can affect your brain and your body, so too can certain foods. Don't worry, I'm not going to give a neurology lecture—I'm just going to provide some basic information that's useful to know.

Although we need to eat to maintain our bodily and mental functions, we've evolved to eat food for more than just survival. We also eat certain foods because of the effect they have on our brains. That's right—simply looking at or thinking about foods you love can activate the area of your brain that is the feel-good section, pleasure area, or reward center. The mere thought of the food can actually trigger the release of a powerful neurotransmitter called dopamine that makes you feel a sense of euphoria.

Don't you believe me when I say that merely thinking about food can affect your body? Try this as a test. Close your eyes and think of a food you love—not just like, but love. How the food smells, what it looks like, and your memory of its taste causes the chemical reaction in the brain I just described. For me, as I write this, I'm thinking of lemon drops—and I kid you not, my mouth is watering! And my body is getting all ready for them.

After you take the first bite, your nervous system goes to work and sends a signal to relax your stomach muscles, which makes you feel like you need to eat more to be satisfied. Your stomach is actually getting bigger and making space for food. At the same time, your taste buds and your nose are producing important feedback signals. So you keep eating more. A classic example is potato chips. We really are wired so that we can't eat just one. Have you ever been able to eat just one chip? I haven't.

Another example of how food affects your brain, which then affects your body, occurs every year on Thanksgiving. Turkey has a lot of tryptophan, an amino acid that is used to produce serotonin. Serotonin helps to induce sleep. So after a big turkey meal, what happens? We often get sleepy.

Food Addiction

I said it before and I need to say it again: if you're overweight, it's not because you lack willpower or are weak. I get very annoyed when I hear people say it's so easy to lose weight. It isn't easy. There are many factors that go into being overweight. Certainly your choice of what you eat is a major factor, but as you have just learned, food can have a significant effect on your brain, which affects how you interact with food. Certain foods have some addictive-like properties, and these can be hard to fight. By no means are you doomed to failure, even if you've tried in the past to lose weight with little success. You just need to know what's going on and figure out how to combat it. It can be a struggle, but you can prevail.

Addiction is a serious matter. I'm not equating addiction to food to addiction to alcohol or drugs, but there are similarities. There are disruptions in the areas of the brain responsible for self-control and pleasure that are seen in food addictions that mirror those in drug addictions. In fact, recent studies have shown through MRIs and CT scans that high-fat, high-sugar food works on the pleasure centers of the brain. When that is the case, your brain wants more of this food to maintain the feeling of pleasure. If you've been eating this food for a while, the body will become used to it, and if you try to stop eating it, your brain will send signals that make you want to eat it—that is, you crave it. Such cravings can be quite powerful.

A craving is a desire for something so strong you *must* have it. For my sister, it's jelly beans—and not just around Easter. There's no adequate substitute for her—not Swedish fish, not licorice, not any other type of candy. She craves jelly beans on a weekly basis, and she makes sure she has them around.

What's going on here? Does she just have a sweet tooth? And if you think about it, why are cravings always for unhealthy foods that are high in fat, such as doughnuts, or high in sugar, like candy? It's never fruit, vegetables, or fish that people crave, is it? I've never met anyone who craves tangerines or sea bass. That's not just a coincidence.

Eating high-sugar or fat-filled foods actually causes chemical reactions in our brains that trigger our bodies to eat more. These chemical reactions make it harder for the body to regulate the appetite. Saturated fats and sugary foods impair the brain's ability to make us realize we are full, until we are stuffed. Before you know it, you've eaten the whole bag of chips or the whole pint of ice cream.

We now know that some foods that are high in sugar increase ghrelin release. High ghrelin stimulates the appetite. So certain foods actually cause chemicals to be released by our brains that in turn cause us to eat more of what we should be eating less of! Fat-filled, sugar-rich foods also increase the levels of opioid receptors in our brains, again giving us pleasure.

Is it a surprise that the average American eats 22.2 teaspoons of sugar each day? This is why it is so hard to fight the cravings. They can be as powerful as narcotics. Your brain has to be rewired. Don't underestimate the power of food on your brain. That's why it is so important to choose carefully what you decide to put in your mouth. And as the research shows, addictions to food are not to be taken lightly. They can impair your quality of life and be deadly like addictions to alcohol and narcotics.

You might find it interesting to learn that drinking lots of calorie-containing liquids (not water, which has no calories) does not trigger the hormones that signal we are full. So we keep drinking calories, and that leads to weight gain. That's why all of those sweet teas and lemonades make you gain a lot of weight; not only are they full of sugar, your brain also doesn't register to your body that you are full despite all of those calories you are drinking. Your brain is thinking, "This tastes good. Give me more." So you keep filling up the glass until the pitcher is empty. The only good news is that water doesn't have calories, so drinking lots of water is fine and actually desirable.

Fighting Cravings

One way to fight your cravings is to outsmart them. Thinking about your craving consumes a lot of mental energy. It makes it hard to think about anything else or even perform your normal daily functions. This is how I am when I am craving coffee in the morning—just ask my wife. But if your brain is otherwise engaged—watching the news, listening to the radio, preparing a report—you'll have fewer brain cells available to be focused on getting the cupcakes you crave.

Another way to rewire the brain and how it interacts with food you want to stop eating is to nip it in the bud. Say you're halfway into a bag of chips. You realize that there is something you can do about it. If you're looking for something crunchy, grab some carrots or celery sticks with all-natural peanut butter or eat a handful of almonds. You can consciously decide to stop eating the bag of chips and replace it with something else. You first have to be aware of why and what you're doing and let your brain work for you. Don't resign yourself to the fact that if you already opened the bag of chips, you have to finish them—or you don't want the ice cream to melt, so you might as well eat the entire carton! You don't need to do either. What you do need to do is to stop kidding yourself.

Don't make it harder on yourself by having the food you're trying to avoid readily available. If the food is close by and there's plenty of it, you're going to eat a bunch. If there are two bags of chocolate chip cookies in your pantry, they are going to be hard to resist. I'm always surprised when patients buy the food they're trying to avoid. I know we all want to be strong, but why test yourself? Don't keep the foods you're trying to avoid in your home.

Phil, one of my patients, is sixty-five years old. He once said to me, "Dr. Whyte, if it's in my house, I will eat it. The way I stopped eating stuff that was bad for me was I quit buying it." Phil has lost nearly forty pounds in the past two years.

I suggest to my patients that they try to keep healthy foods where they can see them and stash the unhealthy ones (if they must have them at all) in a hard-to-reach drawer or cabinet.

Is Occasional Cheating Okay?

Sometimes you should simply give in. That's right—you can cheat. *Occasionally*—that is the key point. I said earlier that this diet is not about denial. I don't want you to never eat something if you truly enjoy it. So if you truly enjoy cupcakes, you should have one every so often—once a week, maybe, but *not* every day. This can actually help you to successfully manage your cravings and thereby control your weight.

Researchers recently learned that desserts like cake and cookies can help dieters to lose more weight and keep it off in the long run—*if* they indulge only occasionally and if they employ some tricks. One trick is to indulge in the morning, when the body's metabolism is revved up; that way, you're better able to work off the extra calories throughout the day. That's much better than eating a slice of your favorite pie late at night.

If you enjoy sweets, I don't want you to avoid them for the rest of your life. That's not what this diet is about, and it's not a good strategy. If you have eaten sweets a lot in the past and now try to avoid them entirely, you might create a psychological craving for them that could lead to bingeing. Eating the unhealthy foods you love occasionally (not more than once a week) can keep cravings under control so they're not as powerful.

Some fad diets are very restrictive in what you can and cannot eat. These often don't work, because you'll actually suffer withdrawal-like symptoms, and most of us will eventually give in. Don't set yourself up for failure. Take small steps on the road to success. This road can include some cheating.

The good news is that eventually you won't even feel like cheating. You won't be interested in and won't crave foods that are not going to help you keep weight off and live longer.

The Magic of Twenty-One Days

Are you familiar with Lent? Many Christians give up something for Lent, which is the forty-day period from Ash Wednesday to Easter. Kids (and even adults) often give up a food they like—it could be candy, brownies, or chocolate, something they really enjoy and would miss but don't really need. A few years ago, I gave up soda. The tough part about Lent is that it lasts so long.

We know from behavioral research that it typically takes about three weeks, roughly twenty-one days, to change a behavior, and that includes fighting food cravings. During the first week, I thought about soda all the time—I walked past a vending machine and often thought, "I'll just give up something else." But I kept at it. Days 3 and 4 weren't much easier. I even had some dreams in which I was drinking soda! I'm serious. By the end of the first week, I had barely made it without drinking soda. I substituted water, which I definitely did not enjoy at first.

During the second week, I wasn't as focused each day on my lack of soda consumption as I was the first week, but it still was a struggle. During the third week, I barely thought of soda at all and was actually enjoying the water; sometimes I had it with a wedge of lime, or sometimes I had sparkling water, which satisfied my need for fizz. And by the fourth week, my thirst for soda was evaporating.

By the time Lent was over, I had no desire to drink a two-liter bottle of soda. Instead, I was enjoying water. And in the last few years, I have probably drunk soda fewer than a dozen times. When I have had it, I felt like it was much too sweet, and I asked myself why I liked it so much. I now drink water at most meals.

This pattern is actually pretty consistent with what we know from neuroscience. It takes three weeks for new brain circuits to form, allowing us to change a behavior. If you can go without something for twenty-one days straight, you will most likely break the link between the food and the desire in the brain.

It's the same for most behaviors. Floss your teeth for twenty-one days straight—no days off—and I bet you'll end up flossing your teeth for most of your life without having to think about it. The key to forming a new habit is to do it for twenty-one days straight—not ten and not fifteen.

Introducing New Foods

There's a similar pattern in introducing new foods to your diet. Too often, people will say, "I don't like broccoli" or "I don't like the taste of skim milk." Research shows that a food has to be introduced to the taste buds thirteen times before the brain and the body can decide if they find the food pleasurable. How many of us give it that many times? Probably very few of us. Try it, and you might be pleasantly surprised.

I had a roommate in medical school who loved whole milk. For a while I tried to convince him that 2 percent or skim milk was much healthier and tasted pretty good. After a considerable amount of my lobbying, he decided to try it. At first, he'd say things like "This tastes like water," but after a week, his attitude was "This isn't so bad." (There was no other type of milk in the house other than 2 percent, so he didn't have much choice.) And by the end of the second week, he actually liked it. When he finally tried whole milk again, he exclaimed, "This tastes like drinking cream!"

I want you to be able to eat foods that you enjoy. And I want to introduce you to some healthy foods that I think you will like. You need to give your body a chance to try them, however, and see if you really like them. Please be open-minded. Don't dismiss certain foods outright because you didn't like them in the past, or worse, because you *think* you won't like them.

I've had many people tell me that they wouldn't like broccoli. When I ask them why, they say, "I just know I wouldn't like it." You can't have that attitude as part of the AARP New American Diet.

Tomatoes are a type of superfood, and I would like you to eat them. But if you try tomatoes thirteen times and still don't like them, I won't force you to eat them.

Stress, Cortisol, and Weight

It's not just the addictive-like properties of food that have your brain and body conspiring against you to prevent you from losing weight. It is also the stress hormone cortisol. I mentioned earlier that your body perceives dieting as starvation and will actually shut down certain body processes to slow your basal metabolic rate and thus lower the expenditure of energy. That way, it makes sure there are more calories going in than calories going out. The hormones leptin and ghrelin keep you hungry and consuming calories. Then cortisol gets into the act by signaling the body to hold on to fat stores.

Cortisol is a hormone that can be very helpful. It provides glucose to the body for energy when there is a stressful situation that requires you to have more energy or to be more alert. But chronic stress will cause your cortisol level to be chronically high, and this is not a good thing for your body. In this situation, the elevated cortisol level causes high blood sugar, which will cause a series of other reactions that will make you store and hold on to fat, so it becomes very difficult to shed the pounds. This explains why stress can actually make you fat.

Meditation and Weight Loss

In recent years, I've been encouraging patients to try meditation, which has been shown to reduce stress. Many people are not initially receptive to the idea. "What about some type of pill instead?" is the usual response! The truth is there are some simple meditation exercises that nearly everyone can do that take only a few minutes.

The focus is on your breathing. The first step is to try to clear your mind of any thoughts. You want to create a sense of calm instead of the constant barrage of thoughts that go through your brain all day.

I suggest you ideally find a quiet place that is comfortable. If you can lie down, do so. But if the only place is your office sitting at your desk, that works, too.

You want to take long, slow breaths. As you inhale, you want to tense your whole body and expand your chest as it fills with air. During this time, you should be focused on your breathing; push out any thoughts that come in your mind. Hold your breath for five to six seconds. You can even count up to six or eight. Then forcibly exhale. Imagine you are throwing your tension and stress away. Repeat this about ten times.

I recommend that people do this at least once a day. This may seem too simple for you, but it can reduce your stress and thereby help you to lose weight.

Ten Steps to Help Your Brain Help You

Now that you understand how your brain responds to food, it's time to give you some tips to help your brain help you to eat a healthier diet:

1. *Be positive.* A positive attitude goes a long way. This isn't Pollyanna mumbo-jumbo, it's based on hard science.

There are certainly going to be ups and downs in your journey to restored health, and you need to believe you can do this. Remember, the mind has a powerful effect on the body, so the first step is believing in yourself, having confidence that you can lose weight and keep it off. If you don't believe you can lose weight, you won't. Sometimes I suggest to people that they picture themselves at the weight they want to be. Or I ask them to find a picture of themselves at a weight they want to get to again. The key is that you have to be positive and envision your new body and healthy lifestyle.

2. *Don't fret setbacks.* Nobody is perfect. You are in this for the long haul. So of course there are going to be setbacks. You're going to binge on ice cream one night after a disagreement with your spouse or an unpleasant review at work. You're going to crave soda and end up drinking it on some days right in the middle of your twenty-one-day plan. It may happen, so don't beat yourself up over it. Just keep moving forward. Remember, you can cheat—just not every day.

3. *Reward yourself for small successes.* Don't wait until you fit into the size 4 dress to consider your changes a success. Instead, reward your behavior, not only the final outcome. Maybe you've gone a week putting vegetables on your plate at every meal. That's a healthy and valuable effort and should be rewarded. Maybe you didn't lose any weight one week, but you didn't gain any, either. Congratulate yourself on the small successes throughout the process. Losing weight and keeping it off is tough work.

4. *Rethink the concept of rewards.* I mentioned earlier that many of us view food as a reward. Instead of always celebrating with food (including those small successes I just mentioned), maybe reward yourself instead with going to the movies or by treating yourself to something at your favorite store, such as a new pair of shoes. This does not mean

that food cannot be part of a celebration, but I want you to rethink the concept that we always celebrate success with huge feasts. This is one of those learned behaviors that we can unlearn.

5. *Try to relieve stress.* There are two big reasons for this. First, if you're an emotional eater, you eat when you're stressed. So the more stressed you are, the more you'll eat. If you can reduce the stress in your life, you'll eat less and then lose more weight. Second, as I mentioned earlier, stress causes cortisol release, which is going to make you store fat. Reduce stress by meditating for a few minutes a day, listening to your favorite music, or taking a five-minute walk to clear your head. Maybe get a ten-minute massage from your loved one. Find what works for you to eliminate some stress in your life.

6. *Get enough sleep.* I write a lot in this book about what you eat, but how much you sleep also determines how much you weigh. Most people don't realize this. We know from numerous studies that not getting enough sleep may lead to weight gain. Sleep benefits many aspects of health, and that includes weight loss. Too many of us dismiss the importance of sleep. It's a key component in your quest to lose weight and keep it off and get healthy. There's no magic amount of sleep that keeps one thin, and sleep needs vary by individual and by age. But we do know this: people who get less than seven hours of sleep a night are more likely to become overweight. If you sleep less than six hours a night, you are 27 percent more likely to become obese. If you sleep a measly four hours a night, you have a 67 percent increased chance of obesity. I recommend seven to nine hours of sleep a night. If you're sleep-deprived, start by increasing sleep by just thirty minutes at a time and slowly build up, so it's not a sudden change. These thirty minutes of extra sleep will give you energy throughout the day, and you'll burn more calories. You also might

want to eat a handful of almonds before you go to bed if you have trouble falling asleep—the tryptophan in the nuts can help you to nod off. And your mother was right in serving you warm milk—it can indeed help you get to sleep.

7. *Don't go to bed too late.* Studies have shown that people who habitually go to bed late (after midnight) and get up late in the morning consume more calories than those who go to bed early and get up early. In some studies, late sleepers were found to eat twice as much fast food and half as many vegetables and fruits than the early risers did. The slogan "Early to bed, early to rise, makes you healthy, wealthy, and wise" should add "and lean." And when you do wake up, open the blinds. There is some good evidence that sunlight boosts the serotonin level, which can elevate your mood and regulate your appetite.

8. *Stop thinking about a diet as denial.* The AARP New American Diet is not about denial. It's about focusing on healthy foods in order to lose weight and live longer. You can't think of losing weight and living longer as a loss of foods you love; remember that your current love of unhealthy foods is a learned behavior. By following the instructions in this book, you will unlearn some old eating habits and learn some new ones. Thinking of everything as denial will ultimately make you resentful, and your body and brain will not respond long-term to the healthy steps you are trying to take. It's about making choices you enjoy that are also healthy.

9. *Develop a support system.* I still remember my seventh-grade teacher, Sister Lady of Fatima, warning us that "birds of a feather flock together." She was basically saying that people hang out with people who are like them. She was also saying that if you hang out with bad characters, people are going to think you're a troublemaker as well. Fast-forward twenty years or so, and the phrase still has meaning. It's important to choose people in your life who are going to

make you a better person. This applies to weight, too. Surround yourself with people who have similar goals or who will at least support your goals. The data show that if most of your friends and/or family members are overweight, you are likely to be overweight. We tend to adopt the eating styles of the people around us. No one wants to be that person who orders a Niçoise salad when everyone else is ordering a steak. So what happens? Everyone orders steaks and fries. But why not be the person who orders the salad? Maybe then everyone else will order a salad.

10. *Ask your family, friends, and colleagues for support.* Just telling people your weight-loss goals often gives you additional motivation to reach them. But I also know that sometimes you don't want to tell people your goals for fear of failing and then possibly being thought less of. The reality is that most of the time, family members and friends are supportive. Tell them what you are trying to do in your desire to become healthy and live longer. Help them to understand why you might be eating different foods or preparing food differently. Positive reinforcement from them can be a key to your success. They may actually join you in your new eating patterns; given the percentage of people who are overweight, they may also wish to lose weight. And don't underestimate the influence of work colleagues. We see and spend more time with our coworkers than we sometimes do with family and friends. Maybe you could even start a walking group at work. Or you could start a stair-climbing group. I know numerous examples of people who have even changed their work environments by getting more fruits and vegetables in the cafeteria and stocking vending machines with healthy options. When you start following the AARP New American Diet, you will be eating differently from many of your friends. But I assure you, it is worth doing. It will take effort, and it will obviously involve real change. So if you can get support from family and friends, do so.

The Importance of Setting Goals

People often ask me whether they should set goals when they are trying to lose weight. I always tell them yes. We know from numerous studies that people who set weight-loss goals more often lose weight than those who have not set goals. For goals to be successful, however, they need to have certain features. I like to see goals that are the following:

- *Realistic.* Too often, patients will be unrealistic in their weight-loss goals. "I'm going to lose fifty pounds by the end of the month" sounds good, but here's the problem: typical weight loss, as well as safe weight loss, is about two or three pounds a week. Knowing that can help you be realistic. And remember, after the initial weight loss in the first few months, it becomes harder to keep losing weight. Choose goals that are manageable changes from the start and that aren't so lofty you'll be overwhelmed. You're in it for a lifetime, so slow and steady is the way to go.

- *Measurable.* If you're going to set goals, you need to measure them. So if your goal is to lose weight, you need to weigh yourself (preferably once a week for the first month and then every week after that). That's pretty straightforward. If your goal is to have more energy to play with your children, then you need to go out on the tennis court or into the backyard and see how long you can play until you need to stop. You need to have a way of measuring your success and compare these measurements over time.

- *Time-sensitive.* To increase your chances of meeting your realistic and measurable goals, you will want to set a deadline. I recommend both short-term and long-term goals. A short-term goal is not "I'm going to lose twenty pounds before the summer" but rather "I'm going to lose two pounds a week for the next four weeks." Short-term goals are usually for less than two months. A long-term goal could be "I'm going to get my blood sugar within a normal range in the next six months." These are general guidelines. I don't want you to set rigid, make-or-break deadlines, since deadlines are typically negative in connotation—meet this deadline or else something bad is going to happen, or if you don't do this you're a failure. The reason both short-term and long-term goals are important is that if you only set long-term goals, you can lose interest in a few weeks or keep pushing off change to the next month. Six months will seem like plenty of time, so often you will delay starting to make changes. Short-term goals will allow you to check on your progress, inspire you to keep moving forward, and let you know when you might need to modify the long-term goals based on your progress, whether good or bad.

- *Actionable.* You have to be able to act on your goals. You can't say, "I'm going to lose weight by running a marathon" if you have a weak knee; you can't act on a goal to drink protein shakes with milk every day if you are lactose-intolerant. You have to choose goals that you can perform some action to reach. And you want to be able to take immediate action. You don't want to wait three months before you can start working toward your goals. It's got to be real change, and you need to be able to start doing it right away.

Sally Changed Her Life for the Better

Sally is a fifty-five-year-old divorced mother of two teenage boys who is also a caretaker for her elderly mother. Sally had been putting on about ten pounds a year for the past two or three years, and she was about twenty-five pounds overweight when she came to see me recently.

Sally was never thin, but usually she was only a few pounds overweight. She had high cholesterol and was borderline diabetic. In the past few years, her life has become more stressful because she got divorced and became primarily responsible for two teenage boys and her mother—all in one house! She told me, "I know why I'm packing on the pounds. I am always on the run—always driving somebody somewhere or picking something up. I eat when I have time and what's around. Fast food gives me more time to juggle more things. I know I don't eat healthy, Dr. Whyte. I've got more important things on my mind."

To help Sally understand the importance of healthy eating as well as the role of stress in her overall health, I made a separate appointment when we could go over how she spent her day and what she ate throughout it. Trying to work this discussion into the standard appointment, when we typically focus on her cholesterol and blood sugar, didn't work. So I decided we needed some dedicated time.

Before our next appointment, I had Sally meet with a dietitian. This presented a great opportunity for her to learn some tips on eating food that is fast and healthy. (After all, you can't get much faster than munching on fruits and vegetables.) She also learned to eliminate most beverages other than water, to eat whole grains instead of processed grains, and to eat more fish and less meat.

When I saw Sally at the next visit, she told me, "Wow, I learned a lot from the dietitian. How come you never told me that stuff?" I chuckled because I *have* given her that information in the past, but not in a separate dedicated appointment that focused only on food. I explained to Sally that eating healthily is actually one of the most important things she can do for herself and her family. Since she is the primary caregiver for her children and her mother, it's important that she maximizes her health. "You can't take care of people if you're sick," I told her.

I also asked about her sleep, specifically about what time she goes to bed, what time she falls asleep, and what time she gets up every day. "Who has time to sleep?" Sally joked. "Seriously, my sleep is lousy. I'm so stressed nowadays about finances and taking care of everyone. I always have something on my mind." I reviewed with her the importance of sleep and how the lack of it can sabotage her weight-loss efforts. "Seriously?" Sally remarked. For the past year, Sally said, she had been sleeping only five to six hours a night—she goes to bed around midnight and is up by six o'clock. Sometimes it takes an hour for her to fall asleep. "There's just not enough time to get everything done," she said. I helped her to understand that her weight gain is not just from the fast-food restaurants and some other unhealthy food choices. It is also due to her stress and her lack of sleep.

I suggested to Sally that she try meditation, especially the meditation techniques that focus on breathing. "I don't have time for that New Age stuff" was her initial response. I went over some simple meditation techniques as well as directed her to some useful websites. Eventually she agreed to try it a couple of times over the next few days.

At her next appointment, we talked about her eating habits, and they had improved. "I feel like I have so much more knowledge on what to eat," she reported. When I asked how the meditation was going, Sally admitted that she really hadn't tried it more than twice. I went over again how the brain affects the body and how stress was most likely making her hold on to weight. She promised me she'd give it another chance. "Maybe I can get my mother to try it with me," she added.

At the next visit, Sally proclaimed, "Those breathing exercises seem to work! My mother and I have been doing them at night, and I am sleeping better. I'm still stressed, but I actually feel it's not as bad." The good news was that with the changes in her diet and her new awareness of the mind-body connection, Sally had lost fifteen pounds within three months of making the changes. A year later, she had lost the entire twenty-five pounds she had gained in the past couple of years.

Two years later, Sally was still eating healthily, still meditating, and still maintaining a normal weight.

Do You Feel More Powerful Now?

By changing your brain's and your body's relationship with food, you will be able to successfully lose weight, live longer, think more clearly, have more energy and vitality, and reduce your risk of various diseases.

6

The AARP New American
Diet Guidelines

In the last five chapters, I've tried to demonstrate to you that what you eat really does matter, that it truly has a profound effect on your health and your life. Now it's time to pull together all of the information I've just given you and create your new diet. Remember, I'm using *diet* as a noun and not a verb. I don't want you to think of this as "I'm dieting." Most overweight people always seem to be dieting but not losing weight or getting healthier. The AARP New American Diet is about healthy eating and maintaining a healthy weight. Through using the research from the NIH-AARP Study as well as other top-notch clinical trials, I've been able to combine the best elements of the Mediterranean diet with the Standard American Diet.

This information concerns making smart food choices backed by the best science. By following the AARP New American Diet, you will lose weight and get healthier because you are eating foods with lots of nutrients. The diet is also tailored to help you reduce your risk of diabetes, heart disease, and cancer by focusing on foods that have been shown to reduce those diseases. And if you already have them, the diet might prevent these conditions from getting worse, improve your quality of life, and help you to live longer.

The diet focuses on foods that will be familiar to you. There are no exotic ingredients that you need to travel miles to find or order online from obscure markets. It is not too complicated, with different things to do on different days of the week. And I'm keeping the directions simple so they will be easy to remember. It can actually be fun to try new foods and cook with different ingredients. You won't get bored with bland food choices in the meals I will describe.

What to Include

The following foods are the main focus of the AARP New American Diet:

- *Vegetables.* Vegetables are a key component of what you should be eating every day. They have everything we discussed: protein, fiber, good carbs, good fats, essential minerals, and vitamins. They are low in calories, yet because of their high water content, they help you to feel full. Because of their texture, they take time to chew, which we know helps to reduce the amount of food we eat. You cannot go wrong by eating a diet that is rich in vegetables.

- *Whole grains.* Whole grains are also a major source of vitamins, minerals, and fiber. They have lots of folate as well, which can be a powerful antioxidant. Because the grain is whole, it contains the germ, endosperm, and bran, compared to refined grains, which contain only the endosperm and have had most of the nutrients stripped away. The bran is important, because it contains some of the B vitamins as well as potassium and magnesium. The germ contains powerful plant oils as well as phytonutrients. The endosperm contains most of the protein, which is good, but all three components are important.

I realize that some diets, such as the primal diet, do not want you to eat whole grains or any grains at all. My training is in health services research—I learned how to study studies and evaluate the evidence. I must tell you I have found no compelling evidence to support the concept that whole grains cause any type of disease. In fact, we know that whole grains actually are quite healthy—they can reduce heart disease, diabetes, and stop some types of cancer, most notably colon cancer. The NIH-AARP Study has consistently shown a health benefit to whole grains. Think about it. Does it really make sense to avoid food that has proven health benefits just because it wasn't eaten two million years ago? Whole grains are an important component of the AARP New American Diet, and this is based on the best science available.

- *Fish.* Fish is another crucial component of the diet. It has the good fats you need, it's low in calories, and it contains important nutrients. Fish has been shown to benefit nearly every part of your body, including your brain. Be aware, though, that some fish contain higher levels of mercury than others, so you should limit your consumption of those types of fish.

- *Fruit.* Fruit is Mother Nature's candy. Some fad diets foolishly discourage eating fruit, but I encourage it. Fruit is a great source of fiber. Remember that high-fiber foods help you to lose weight because they make you feel fuller on fewer calories. Fruit is also high in important vitamins and minerals. It is true that fruit has sugar, and that's why some diets discourage it. The reality is, however, that the body responds to the natural sugar found in fruit differently from the highly processed sugars found in foods such as pastries and candy. The old adage "An apple a day keeps the doctor away" has a lot of science behind it.

- *Low-fat dairy.* Please don't dismiss dairy. Dairy products, including low-fat milk, cheese, and yogurt, are important. Many women will say they don't drink milk because it is too fattening. Milk does have fat and sugar, but it also has protein and numerous health benefits. Choose the low-fat variety, and you will be fine. Dairy is a rich source of calcium and vitamin D, which we know many women and some men do not get enough of. So it's important to consume dairy products. Most of us should probably increase our dairy consumption, especially as we get older, since we need the bone-building calcium and protective effects of vitamin D. Remember, though, that dairy, for our purposes, does not include ice cream. Some people are lactose-intolerant, so check out dairy alternatives or take a lactase pill before consuming milk products.

  I realize that some diets discourage you from consuming dairy products. This includes the primal diet as well as some others. The primal diet excludes dairy because animals had not yet been domesticated (and were therefore not milked) in the hunter-gatherer era. Other diets exclude it because they are concerned about the fat content and calories.

  If you choose low-fat dairy products, you consume little saturated fat, and the number of calories is relatively small and worth the health benefit. This includes reducing your risk of heart disease and diabetes. You are much better off consuming low-fat dairy than fruit juices and simple sugars. Several studies have shown that people who consume three servings of low-fat dairy a day lose more weight over time than those who consume one or none.

- *Nuts.* Nuts are a great source of protein and healthy fats. They are low in volume but can help you to feel full. They are probably the most underrated and underused foods of a weight-loss and healthy living plan, but they should be eaten in moderation.

These food groups are the most important components of the AARP New American Diet. We know from the NIH-AARP Study that these foods will improve your health and help you to lose weight—the purpose of this book!

What to Exclude

What you exclude from your diet is as important as what you include. So don't just add the food groups discussed above to what you currently eat; you also need to exclude, or at least cut back as much as possible on, the following types of foods:

- *Highly processed foods.* When food is processed and refined, it's a bad thing. Processing causes the food to lose most if not all of its nutrient value. It can be misleading when you see the word *enriched* on a package. The reality is that these "enriched" foods are typically not as nutritious as the nonprocessed alternative. This applies to all the food groups, whether it's grains, meat, vegetables, or fruit. In general, most food that comes in packages is processed. This doesn't mean you can't have any processed foods, but the less you have, the better.

- *High-sugar foods.* I'm not sure where to start in listing the problems with high-sugar foods. The list would go on and on. One of the biggest problems is that sugary foods are low in nutrients. In addition, a high amount of sugar basically acts like a toxin in our bodies, causing problems with insulin release and fat deposits.

- *Saturated fat.* Some of the strongest data for heart disease and cancer are related to saturated fat. The biggest culprit is meat; not only is it typically high in saturated fat; it is also low in volume and high in calories. We tend to eat a lot of it—just ask my teenage nephew, who seems to be able to eat several hamburgers in just ten minutes.

Out of Sight, Out of Mind

Now that you know the general principles, how do you make them part of your daily life? The first step is to clean out your kitchen and pantry. Consider this similar to spring cleaning. Just as you empty your closets of items you no longer need or want, this is the time to empty the house of foods you no longer want to eat or should eat.

I'm going to change the classic phrase "out of sight, out of mind" to "out of sight, out of mind, out of mouth." This really does work. We have already covered the topic of the brain-body-food connection. Why tempt yourself with food that is unhealthy, has no nutrients, and makes you gain weight and develop disease? We've cut through the clutter; you are no longer kidding yourself, so now it's time to make a real change.

What needs to go? I think you know by now. You need to ditch the following:

- Soda—both diet and regular
- Full-fat dairy
- Sports drinks
- Fruit drinks (including juices and especially blends)
- Energy drinks
- Lemonade
- Cakes, including cupcakes, cheesecake, crumb cake, coffee cake, and brownies
- Cake mixes
- Cake frosting
- Pastries made with white flour, including muffins, doughnuts, scones, biscotti, and biscuits
- White-flour bagels
- Chips, including potato chips, corn chips, salsa chips, tortilla chips, dipping chips, and nachos
- Crackers
- Cookies
- Cheese dips
- White rice
- White sugar
- Candy of any type
- Salad dressings, except low-fat, low-sugar, and vinaigrette
- Soy sauce
- Ice cream
- Instant oatmeal (the sweetened, flavored kind)
- Highly processed cereals (including anything that says "fruit flavored")

- White pasta, including macaroni and cheese
- Processed meats, including lunch meats, bacon, hot dogs, salami, bologna, pastrami, pepperoni, sausage, and ham
- Corn
- White bread and rolls
- Beer
- Mixers for alcohol
- Hard liquor
- Butter
- Margarine
- Cooking spray
- Artificial sweeteners
- White potatoes, including instant (sweet potatoes are okay)
- Instant noodles
- Canned soup
- Peanut butter (unless all-natural)
- Jelly of any kind
- Rice cakes
- Anything that includes high-fructose corn syrup or partially hydrogenated oil in the ingredients list (These are connected with numerous health conditions, such as diabetes, cancer, obesity, heart disease, allergies, asthma, and they might accelerate the aging process.)

I'm sure getting rid of these was hard to do, and you probably struggled with quite a few items on the list. I bet you even kept a few—and that's okay. Remember, this is not about denial, so if you really want a hot dog every once in a blue moon, that's fine. If you really crave a piece of pizza, go for it occasionally, but also add a salad with vegetables. Instead of eating ice cream at night, consider an all-natural sorbet or a frozen banana. I truly believe that as you change your eating patterns and understand the power of food, you simply won't want the unhealthy foods you liked in the past. You'll be asking yourself, "Do I really want to eat that?"

Build It and They Will Come

The next step is to restock your kitchen and pantry. Stock up on healthy foods that are filled with nutrients. I encourage you to buy in large quantities. Going shopping on the weekends works for most people so they are not rushed. Do not go grocery shopping while you're hungry—that's a sure recipe for disaster. Every sugary and salty food will be calling out your name and tempting you to put it in your cart.

When you go shopping, focus on the edges of the store—that's where you'll find the fruits and vegetables. If you start there, you won't forget to include them. It's also where stores keep most of the healthy unprocessed food—and it's the area that you probably spent the least amount of time in. That is, until now!

Too often, we simply eat what's available. And up to now, it was probably unhealthy food that was available. If you're hungry and there are only potato chips around, I can understand that this is what you ate. But now you know better. Focus on the following:

- Whole-wheat pasta
- Whole-grain whole wheat bread, whole-grain rye bread, whole-grain pumpernickel, and whole-grain oat bread
- Whole-wheat pita pockets and tortillas
- Whole oats
- Whole-wheat crackers
- Seeded crackers
- Whole-wheat flour
- Whole-wheat pizza crust
- Whole-grain cereal
- Brown rice
- Couscous
- Quinoa
- Low-fat milk
- Low-fat cottage cheese
- Low-fat string cheese
- Greek yogurt
- Unsalted nuts, such as walnuts, almonds, pistachios, peanuts, cashews, and pine nuts
- Eggs
- Salad greens
- Spinach
- Avocados
- Tomatoes (including canned)
- Carrots
- Celery
- Garlic
- Onions (red and yellow), shallots, scallions, and leeks

- Zucchini and yellow squash
- Brussels sprouts
- Cucumbers
- Beets
- Radishes
- Broccoli
- Cauliflower
- Mushrooms
- Cabbage
- Green beans
- Asparagus
- Bell peppers
- Eggplant
- Artichokes
- Winter squash
- All-natural peanut butter and other natural nut butters
- Raisins
- Unsweetened cranberries
- Bananas
- Cherries
- Grapes
- Apples
- Kiwi
- Pears
- Grapefruit
- Tangerines and oranges
- Raspberries, blueberries, blackberries, and strawberries
- Watermelon and cantaloupe
- Mangoes
- Figs
- Herbs and spices, such as parsley, oregano, black pepper, rosemary, and thyme
- Vanilla extract
- Vinaigrette and natural low-fat, low-sugar salad dressings
- Coffee
- Beans, such as lentils, black beans, kidney beans, and garbanzo beans
- Vinegar
- Lemons and limes
- Flaxseed
- Canned tuna
- Fish, such as salmon, tuna, tilapia, halibut, and mackerel
- Carved fresh turkey
- Chicken breast
- Rotisserie chicken
- Lean red meat
- Canola oil and olive oil
- Olives
- Hummus

Fresh, Frozen, or Canned?

Many people want to know if it really matters whether fruits and vegetables are fresh, frozen, or canned. Is fresh always better? It's a great question; the answer is that it depends.

In general, I would prefer that you choose fresh fruits and vegetables over canned or frozen. Depending on the season and where you live, however, that may not always be possible. I would rather that you eat frozen or canned fruits and vegetables than none at all.

Most people don't realize that sometimes canned and frozen fruits and vegetables have more nutrients than fresh ones. That's because they are canned and frozen at the peak of freshness, when they are packed with nutrients. Some of these nutrients are lost in the preservation process, but canned and frozen produce can be more nutritious than fruit and vegetables that are over the hill. Sometimes salt is added to canned products, so you should look at the sodium content and choose low-sodium versions. Sugar is also often added, so avoid sugar-sweetened canned goods. If the fruits and vegetables are picked before they are ripe, they will not have formed all of the nutrients that they would have if they had been allowed to ripen. And if you buy fresh and don't eat it for a while, it's going to go bad and will be a waste of money.

The bottom line is that I want you to eat more fruits and vegetables—and it doesn't matter that much whether they are fresh, frozen, or canned.

Healthy Food Is Not Necessarily More Expensive

Over the years, I have had many people tell me that they cannot eat healthy food because it's just too expensive. The reality is that with all of the food choices we have today, healthy food is quite affordable.

A recent study by the U.S. Department of Agriculture (USDA) found that foods like milk, yogurt, carrots, bananas, beans, and coffee are less expensive than common unhealthy foods like cinnamon buns, doughnuts, bagels, hot dogs, and soda. One reason people assume junk food is more affordable is that the cost comparisons done in the past used a cost-per-calorie measurement. Since vegetables and fruits don't have as many calories, they would appear to be more expensive per calorie. Foods that contain a lot of sugar and saturated fat have a lot of calories, so they would be perceived as cheaper. But remember, the AARP New American Diet is not about counting calories.

When looking at portion sizes, the USDA found that the cheapest food to eat is grains, followed by dairy, vegetables, and fruit. The key when determining your grocery budget is to consider the entire cost of your diet—and that includes not only the cost of your meals but also the cost of your health.

Hide Unhealthy Foods You Still Like

Now that you have restocked your kitchen and pantry, here's one of the best pieces of advice. I know some of you are still keeping foods around that I would prefer you exclude. So the way to handle this is to put the healthy foods right in the front of the refrigerator and on the middle pantry shelves. That way, when you go looking for food, they will be the first things you'll see. If you make it harder to find the foods you want to give up, that extra time might allow you to change your mind and instead make a healthier and smarter choice.

The AARP New American Diet "Instead of" List

Over the years, I've learned that it helps to give specific advice early in a weight-loss plan. Again, I want to make this simple for you, so I've created an "Instead of" list. I have identified items that you might have been eating, and I am gently suggesting a healthier option. Here are some ideas:

- Choose brown rice *instead of* white rice.
- Choose whole-wheat bread *instead of* white bread.
- Choose whole-wheat pasta *instead of* regular pasta.
- Choose sweet potatoes *instead of* white potatoes.
- Choose figs *instead of* sugary cookies.
- Choose a handful of almonds *instead of* a candy bar.
- Choose unbuttered popcorn *instead of* potato chips.
- Choose a small bowl of Greek yogurt *instead of* ice cream.
- Choose grilled or roasted chicken *instead of* fried chicken.
- Choose unsalted whole-wheat pretzels *instead of* regular pretzels.
- Choose four ounces of broiled salmon *instead of* fried fish sticks.
- Choose high-fiber, low-sugar cereal *instead of* sugary cereal.
- Choose steel-cut oats or rolled oats *instead of* instant oatmeal with added sugar.
- Choose a handful of blueberries *instead of* a candy bar.
- Choose nuts or seeds *instead of* chips or crackers.
- Choose all-natural nut butters for toast and bread *instead of* regular butter.
- Choose olive oil *instead of* butter for cooking.
- Choose oil and vinegar *instead of* prepared salad dressing.
- Choose a small piece of dark chocolate *instead of* a milk chocolate candy bar.
- Choose a whole chicken or turkey and slice it up *instead of* processed lunch meats.
- Choose a frozen banana *instead of* a chocolate milk shake.

Advice for Meat Lovers

I realize that many of you enjoy meat, so it's not realistic to suggest that you don't eat it at all. As you'll see, I want you to reduce what types of meat you eat, how much, and how often. If you are going to eat meat, it is important to choose lean meats such as skinless chicken, pork tenderloin, and loin roast. You should avoid frequent consumption of beef, lamb, and venison, since they are high in saturated fat.

When you do eat red meat, look at the cut. I've learned over time that the redder, the better. The marbling is actually fat. It may make the meat tasty, but you'll learn other ways to bring out the flavor of meat. When you cook the meat, trim away much of the white fat. When buying ground beef, choose 85 to 90 percent lean. Look for extra-lean cuts: eye of round roast, top round steak, tenderloin, bottom round roast, and top sirloin steaks.

For poultry, choose the white meat. I remember when I was growing up, everyone would fight for the leg. Do you still? Well, don't pick that fight—choose white pieces over dark. White meat contains fewer calories and less saturated fat than dark meat.

• •

AARP New American Top Twenty-Five Diet Busters and Boosters

Top Twenty-Five Diet Busters

1. Skipping breakfast
2. Eliminating low-fat dairy
3. Eating too fast
4. Drinking diet soda
5. Never cheating
6. Eating out-of-control portions
7. Eating out more than three times a week
8. Drinking fewer than six glasses of water a day
9. Drinking alcohol more than three days a week

10. Eliminating carbs
11. Sleeping less than six hours a night
12. Drinking sweetened high-fat specialty coffees
13. Never weighing yourself
14. Filling up with bread
15. Eating red meat more than four days a week
16. Automatically choosing low-fat food
17. Avoiding fruit, especially berries
18. Eating after eight o'clock at night
19. Overestimating how many calories are burned by exercise
20. Eliminating snacking
21. Failing to reduce stress
22. Drinking sports drinks
23. Choosing "diet foods" for your meals
24. Eating granola bars
25. Counting calories

Top Twenty-Five Diet Boosters

1. Eating slowly, taking at least thirty minutes for a meal
2. Chewing sugar-free gum
3. Cheating once a week
4. Consuming low-fat dairy
5. Drinking two cups of caffeinated coffee a day
6. Sleeping at least seven hours a night
7. Meditating a few minutes every day
8. Eating a handful of nuts every day
9. Eating fish instead of meat two or three times a week
10. Eating a piece of fruit every day
11. Consuming a handful of berries every day
12. Eating smaller meals, more often
13. Exercising for at least thirty minutes three days a week
14. Weighing yourself once a week

15. Drinking a glass of water before each meal
16. Eliminating white bread
17. Reducing the amount of processed food consumed
18. Eating oatmeal or Greek yogurt for breakfast
19. Eating at a table with your food on a plate
20. Avoiding vending machines
21. Never saying "supersize"
22. Using olive oil for cooking
23. Sharing a dessert
24. Getting rid of the salt shaker (see chapter 7)
25. Eating a quarter ounce of dark chocolate daily

• •

Bob Loves Butter

Bob is a sixty-five-year-old widower. He lives alone; his two grown children reside across the country. Bob recently learned to cook, and he enjoys it.

Bob has never been thin. When I started working with him, he was about forty pounds overweight and had high blood pressure and high cholesterol, both being treated with medications. He had a heart attack about five years ago.

I have often talked to Bob about his weight. Since he prepares his food himself, I told him that he largely can control his weight by what food he cooks, as well as how he cooks it. "Have you considered using olive oil?" I asked him recently.

"Nah, I'm old-school," he replied. "I use butter; it gives food flavor. Everything can taste good with butter. Besides, isn't olive oil what the snooty French use to cook? I don't like French food." I explained to Bob that some of the best chefs use olive oil to cook. He didn't seem interested in that. "I'll never be a great chef," he stated.

I pointed out that olive oil could provide a new taste for him, and he did agree to try new foods; he seemed mildly interested in that. Finally, I pointed out that olive oil has healthy fats, whereas the butter he uses to cook is an unhealthy fat. If he switched from butter to olive oil, I said, I might be able to lower the dosage of his cholesterol medication. And it might even protect him from future heart damage. That got his attention! "You know I don't like being on pills, Dr. Whyte," he said. "I can give that olive oil a try."

At his next visit three months later, Bob commented, "That olive oil isn't so bad. Things cook pretty fast with it, and it's not a bad taste." From Bob, that's a compliment. I provided him with some ideas on how to use olive oil in salads. He said he'd give it a try.

"So can I come off the meds yet?" was his main question for me. His cholesterol numbers were the same— not any better, not any worse. I asked him how often he used olive oil instead of butter. He confessed that he had used it only two or three times a week. I suggested he switch to olive oil exclusively instead of butter and focus on eating more vegetables.

Four months later, Bob had lost twelve pounds, and his cholesterol level was almost normal. "You know, Dr. Whyte, that butter seemed to make me eat so much more food," he said. "With the olive oil, I've actually cut down on portion sizes. And I even enjoy the occasional salad with olive oil and nuts."

"Wow!" I exclaimed, adding jokingly, "Planning a trip to Paris anytime soon?"

"Nah, I like it here," he replied.

A year later, Bob had lost an additional fifteen pounds and was able to go off his cholesterol medications.

7

The Meal Plans:
7, 14, and 30 Days

In the last six chapters, I've shared quite a bit of science about nutrition and health. Now it's time to put that information into practice. The AARP New American Diet meal plans are broken down into three parts: a 7-day plan, a 14-day plan, and a 30-day plan. I have included a variety of different foods, some of which will be new to you. I encourage you to try new foods, new combinations of foods you already eat, and new methods of cooking.

In order to lose weight and become healthier, you will need to adopt new and different ways of eating. After each week, I will ask you to do a check-in on your weight, your BMI, and your waist circumference. The key to success will be to keep the entire plan in mind, but to take it one day at a time.

The First Two Weeks

I promised to take the guesswork out of this diet and make it easy to follow. So here's what I want you to do for the first two weeks:

1. *Drink water*. Water is one of the two beverages you may drink during the first two weeks; the other is coffee. Water is naturally filling—unlike some other liquids, water can stretch your stomach, and that sends signals to your brain that you are full, even though water has no calories. Water aids in digestion, allowing your body to absorb nutrients more effectively. And drinking water during a meal keeps your mouth busy, so it takes you longer to eat. Since we know that it can take twenty minutes for our brains to register that we are full, the longer we take to eat, the less food we'll consume, protecting us from overeating. Studies have shown that people who drink two cups of water before each meal eat 40 percent less calories throughout the day than those who don't drink water before eating. By taking this advice, you'll actually feel fuller on less food.

2. *Drink* lots *of water*. There are actually some data that low daily water consumption—fewer than two glasses a day— may increase the blood sugar level, predisposing some people to diabetes. We're not exactly sure why this is the case, but it might be because people are choosing sugary beverages like soda or energy drinks that lead to weight gain and weaken the body's control of blood sugar. So the healthiest choice is always going to be water. Drink up, preferably six to eight glasses a day. Don't wait until you're thirsty to drink; by that time you are already down a quart of water. When your body is fully hydrated, it seems to burn more calories as a result of a faster-functioning metabolism—an added benefit of being well hydrated.

3. *Drink coffee*. Coffee is the other beverage you may drink during the first two weeks. As I've said, the NIH-AARP Study points to the health benefits of coffee. Too often,

coffee has gotten a bum rap. The reality is that coffee is healthier to drink than most other beverages, including tea. (Although research points to certain health benefits of tea, there are not as much data supporting tea drinking as there are for coffee drinking.) The key is that no sugar or artificial sweeteners are allowed; adding low-fat milk, however, is allowed. Please note that when I say to drink coffee, I do not mean all those specialty sweetened coffee drinks. Plain coffee doesn't have any calories, but specialty coffee usually does. Some lattes and especially frappuccinos can have as many calories as a fast-food hamburger—so only regular coffee, please. I'd prefer that you drink caffeinated coffee, but decaf will do.

4. *Avoid fruit juice.* People often ask me if fruit juice is okay to drink. Fruit juices and vitamin waters do have some benefits, but overall, water is still the better choice, and that's the choice I'd like you to make exclusively early on (except for coffee). No sugar-sweetened tea or lemonade. No sports drinks, either, weekend athletes.

5. *Avoid soda.* The AARP New American Diet is a strict no-soda diet, and that includes diet soda. Most Americans drink about two sodas a day, so replacing sugary soda with water can save more than three hundred calories a day. Replacing all beverages with water would save more than six hundred calories a day. Even at half of that rate, you could lose twenty-five pounds in a year simply by eliminating soda.

6. *Consider carbonating your water.* One way to help you eliminate your desire for soda yet still follow the water-only rule is to make your own soda. Sometimes people simply enjoy the fizz of soda, and nowadays you can make your own fizz. There are lots of devices you can buy that will provide carbonation to water. My wife loved the lime soda we used to buy at our local grocery store. We weren't surprised to learn that it had more sugar in it than regular soda. So I convinced her to buy a carbonation device, and now she

makes her own lime soda with lime juice and water—it has fizz and nearly zero calories. Unsweetened flavored seltzers are also fine for this diet, and of course, you can buy bottled carbonated water.

7. *Avoid alcohol.* During the first two weeks, I also want you to eliminate alcohol. I realize that the Mediterranean diet includes red wine, but alcohol, including red wine, has a high number of calories. Right now I want you to reduce your total calorie consumption, and an easy way to do that is to eliminate all calories from liquids—and that includes alcohol.

8. *Avoid white grains.* Eliminate any food that is white unless it's low-fat dairy. I'm overgeneralizing a little, but by this I basically mean products made from white flour, including bread, pasta, pastries, and cakes, as well as white rice. These are processed grains, which I want you to avoid because they are one of the main causes of obesity and subsequent disease. To help you remember: "If it's white, it's not right."

9. *Avoid potatoes.* Avoid potatoes during this period. I know many of you have grown up with white potatoes as a common staple, and they're an example of something we thought was healthy but probably isn't. A recent study found that for every serving per day of potatoes, people gained nearly two pounds a year; obviously, potato chips and french fries caused even more weight gain. So for the first two weeks, potatoes and all potato derivatives should be avoided.

10. *Avoid sugar.* Do not add sugar to anything—including your coffee, oatmeal, or cereal. This includes not only granulated sugar but also confectioner's sugar, brown sugar, honey, maple syrup, molasses, regular corn syrup, and high-fructose corn syrup.

11. *Eat breakfast every day.* This means a *real* breakfast, not a bagel and coffee. If you replace eating no breakfast with

eating a breakfast of highly processed simple carbs, you're just exchanging one bad habit for another. I'm going to give you some specific breakfast recipes to make this easy, but you should know that you might need to get up a few minutes earlier to prepare it and eat it. Believe me, it is worth it. Many people will say they are not hungry in the morning; I was like that for a long time. I barely ate anything and was always in a rush to get to the office. So I started with something small, like two pieces of whole-wheat toast, and then over a few days I built up to a variety of fruit, yogurt, fiber cereal, and eggs. Now I almost never leave home without taking the time to eat breakfast. Eating a healthy, nutrient-dense breakfast is probably one of the best changes you can make to ensure success; it will keep your blood sugar and insulin levels steady all morning. If you're consistently hungry by late morning, it's because you aren't eating enough first thing in the morning.

12. *Eat more often.* Not only will you need to eat breakfast every day, but you'll also need to eat more frequently. On the surface, it may sound like skipping a meal is a good way to reduce your caloric intake. But that just makes you hungrier later on, and you're likely to consume more calories than you would have done by eating a good hearty breakfast, lunch, or dinner. I want you to eat three small meals a day and have at least one midmorning or afternoon snack. Ideally, I want you to eat five times a day, and I'll be showing you how to do that. Eating more often gets your metabolism going and burns more calories, so believe it or not, eating more frequently will often result in weight loss! Lots of research has shown that if you eat smaller meals more often, you won't get as hungry. Think about it—if you are waiting six to eight hours between meals, by the time you're able to eat, you are going to eat a lot of food and therefore consume a lot of calories. It has happened to me, and I'm sure it has happened to you. On a long car trip, by the time you finally make a pit stop, I bet you eat a lot more

food than you normally would—you are famished and basically inhale a couple of burgers, a large order of french fries, and a big soda. At that point, even the beef jerky is looking pretty good! Eating smaller meals more frequently will prevent that intense hunger. The AARP New American Diet encourages smart snacking.

Shift more of your calories to the first half of the day, when you still have time to burn them off, rather than the second half of the day, which is when most of us eat more. When you eat is as important as what you eat. Too much food—even if it's healthy food—in the second half of the day will cause you to gain weight. It would be great if your biggest meal was in the morning and you ate less and less at each subsequent meal. I know that's not necessarily realistic, but you can at least shift the burden of calories to earlier in the day.

13. *Eat fish.* Eat a serving of fish at least twice, ideally three times, a week instead of meat. Fish is naturally low in saturated fat. This will probably be a big change for you, since the Standard American Diet focuses on meat and potatoes. The Mediterranean diet focuses on fish and vegetables. Remember, this is about *substituting* fish for meat. Sometimes women give up meat in the belief that they are giving up calories, but then instead of choosing fish, they eat heavy cheese or high-calorie, refined carbs such as pasta and bread. Fish really is key here, and there are many types to choose from. Try different ones to find the types you enjoy.

14. *Avoid eating out.* Eating out is fraught with danger. It's very hard to stick with your new way of eating when you have less control over the content of the food and how it's prepared. This limitation is only for the first two weeks. After that, you'll be more knowledgeable and further along in your new way of eating so that you'll be better equipped to make good choices. I don't want you to have to tackle too much too soon, so stay home, where you can be in complete control of what you put in your mouth.

Some Tools to Help You

There are also a few other tools I'd like you to try. They might seem a little kooky, but there are good data to support them:

1. *Chew sugar-free gum.* Chewing gum does not require a lot of energy, but it releases two hormones that may signal your brain that you are full. Therefore, when you do eat a meal or a snack, you will eat less. Chewing gum also helps if you're a nibbler; it keeps you from nibbling food as you cook it, eating chips while you're watching TV, or mindlessly grazing on salty or sugary snacks while you're surfing the Web. Chewing sugar-free gum also helps to reduce cavities, and improving your oral health can actually improve the health of your heart.

2. *Eat at a table.* There are a couple of reasons for sitting at a table to eat. You'll eat more slowly, which will give your brain the chance to signal your body that you are full. Data show that when people eat at a table, rather than sitting in their car or standing up, they eat less. Some dietitians even use the phrase "plate, chair, table" to remind you of this technique.

3. *Control your portion sizes.* Realize what portion sizes should look like for weight loss versus how they have been for you. I have no doubt that you need to reduce the amount of food you eat, and one of the easiest ways to do this is to reduce the size of your portions. You have probably heard about different techniques for remembering what a portion size should be. Some good examples are that fruit and vegetable portions should be the size of your fist, a piece of meat should be no bigger than a deck of cards, and a piece of fish should be the size of a checkbook. Portions of whole grains can be the size of two Ping Pong balls.

   I also recommend that you consider using smaller bowls, plates, and eating utensils. Believe it or not, people who do this eat less. And when you do use that plate, make sure half of it is covered with vegetables. I know a lot of households serve food "family style," and I am all about the family. But the problem is that when food is served on large platters, people tend to keep filling up their individual plates. So if they see more pasta left in the bowl or more chicken cutlets on a platter, they think, "I might as well have a little more. I don't want it to go to waste," and then they end up eating more than they should. So for the first two weeks, please don't serve food family style—or if you do, take just one reasonable portion.

4. *Don't count calories or calculate percentages.* Turning your meals into a mathematical calculation is neither realistic nor practical. But another reason not to do this is that some dieters get good at it and buy a lot of packaged food that has the information they are looking for. And packaged food typically has the bad carbs, bad fats, and poor proteins I'm trying to get you to avoid. This isn't always the case, but don't feel pressured to do math that makes you buy food that is packaged.

5. *Don't eat after eight o'clock at night.* Nighttime noshing has to go. Why? We are less active at night, so we burn fewer calories, and instead of losing weight, we pack on the pounds. Remember to try to shift most of your calories to the first half of the day from the second half of the day. If you are hungry at night, it might be because you're eating dinner too early. For instance, if you eat dinner at five and are hungry again at nine, move your dinner to six-thirty, and that will probably solve the problem. I also find that it's not so much the lateness that's the issue; it's probably what you're eating at that time. Most of the time when people eat late at night, it's the high-fat, high-sugar foods that are typically so addictive. The sooner you eliminate nighttime eating, the sooner you will lose weight.

6. *Avoid vending machines.* I know that some vending machines have gotten healthier options in recent years, but they are still pretty dreadful. You definitely don't want your food

choices limited by what's available. Instead, you need to plan your meals, including your smart snacking foods, the night before so you're not in a situation where you're dependent on the choice of chips versus cookies. There have been times when I wished I had some celery and all-natural peanut butter—but if I don't plan it, the licorice in the vending machine looks pretty good.

Too many people use the excuse that they can't stick to a diet because they're hungry all the time. The simple fact is they just aren't eating the right foods and aren't using the right tools to help their brains to signal their bodies that they are full.

Cooking Methods Matter

How you prepare foods goes a long way in determining both how healthy they are and whether you will like them. Check the quality of your utensils. For instance, use a nonstick skillet if you don't already; this will eliminate the need for unhealthy oils or butter to prevent foods from sticking. You could also use an "oil-o-pump," which is like a mister. You place olive oil or canola oil in a bottle that functions as a pump. You spray the oil onto the pan and thus avoid all the unnatural substances in cooking sprays.

Just as I suggested an "instead of" approach for food in the previous chapter, I'm now going to give you an "instead of" approach for cooking:

- Choose lemon juice, herbs, and spices *instead of* salt.
- Choose olive oil (preferably extra-virgin) *instead of* butter or vegetable oil for cooking.
- Choose canola oil *instead of* corn oil.
- Choose broiling, baking, or grilling *instead of* frying.

Be sure not to overcook vegetables, because too much heat will destroy the vitamins and minerals that are so abundant in this food group. Overcooking also destroys the texture and the taste that I think many of you enjoy.

What about Coconut Oil?

Coconut oil has been in the news lately, and many patients as well as friends have asked me whether it's healthy. Some dietitians even suggest that it can help you lose weight. Should you be cooking in it and maybe even adding it to foods?

Let's review what coconut oil is. Coconut oil is made from the dried fruit of the coconut tree. The big concern about coconuts and coconut oil is that it contains a lot of fat and therefore a lot of calories. One tablespoon has more than a hundred calories and more than twelve grams of fat, at least 90 percent of it saturated.

The theory for weight loss is that coconut oil revs up your metabolism and burns calories, perhaps by improving your thyroid output. But the data have been mixed. Some small studies have shown benefits, but other studies have shown either no benefits or some harm. I don't think the high number of calories and the high amount of saturated fat are good for you, so until there are better studies, I say save the coconut oil for when you're on vacation in a tropical paradise. We already have better options for cooking, such as extra-virgin olive oil. Sticking with what we know rather than using what is still being studied has better health benefits.

Eating Out

When I said earlier that you shouldn't eat out for the first two weeks, I didn't mean just in restaurants; it also includes going to other people's homes. But at the very least, avoid eating in restaurants and fast-food establishments, because they can quickly make you veer off your path to weight loss and a healthier you.

One reason for this is that restaurant portions tend to be large. There are some estimates that serving sizes in restaurants are three times what is normally served at home. Restaurants keep portions larger without going bankrupt by using lower-quality meats and processed foods that often have lots of bad fats. Another reason is that they use cooking methods with oils and butters that aren't healthy. Lots of fat and salt is added for flavor, and it makes you feel full—so you feel you got what you paid for.

After the first two weeks, I know you will be eating out at least occasionally, and that's fine. Here are eight tips to bring the AARP New American Diet on the road when you head out of the house to a restaurant:

1. Know the following buzzwords and avoid dishes prepared these ways, because they will have too many calories that aren't worth it: *fried* (especially *deep-fried*), *crispy, battered, breaded, au gratin, alfredo,* and *creamy.*

2. Look for these buzzwords and gravitate toward dishes prepared these ways: *grilled, steamed, broiled,* and *poached.*

3. Do not drink alcohol at the bar while you wait for a table—alcohol has too many calories and can increase the risk of health problems. And all of those salty snacks are going to make you thirsty for more alcohol (which will in turn make you even more thirsty, since alcohol acts as a diuretic), which will make you drink more alcohol, and so on—you get the point. Instead, order water or club soda with lemon or lime and stand away from the bar.

4. Choose an entrée from the appetizer section. Instead of supersizing, which causes you to eat more, downsize so you'll eat less. Portions of appetizers are smaller and may often make more sense. Some dietitians suggest that you order from the children's menu, but honestly, those dishes usually aren't healthier options, so there's no need to go there.

5. Tell the waiter not to bring bread. I always do that. Bread is the number one source of sodium. And whenever there is bread at the table, I bet you eat it and then eat some more. It's amazing behavior to watch. A server puts a plate down and often doesn't even say anything, and we automatically start eating it. It's Pavlovian. Again, it's a learned behavior that you can unlearn. The exception is if it's whole-wheat or rye bread, which it rarely is. Ever wonder why that is?

6. Ask questions. I know there was a time when waiters and waitresses used to get annoyed when people asked question or made substitutions. And I'm sure they still do at some places. But don't be afraid to ask whatever you want. You aren't there to make friends—you're there to get a good, healthy meal. Nowadays, more people are asking good questions: How is it prepared? Can you not add any salt? Can you substitute fruit? Remember, you're paying for the meal—they're not giving it to you for free, so speak up. You can even ask to have your food prepared a certain way—there is a kitchen, after all. I ask questions all the time. Many restaurants are trying to offer healthier choices; for instance, at some Asian restaurants, you can get brown rice instead of white rice. You usually just have to ask. Don't be timid. This is your health we are talking about!

7. Always ask for dressings and sauces on the side. These are two major sources of unhealthy and nutrient-poor calories. By having them put on the side, you can add them sparingly to your salad or entrée.

8. Sharing is caring. If you really need to have a dessert, compromise by sharing it with one or more of the people you're eating with. This way you can still have a few bites to enjoy, but you won't consume all of the calories you normally would by eating it all yourself. Sharing will also help to keep the bill low!

What about Salt?

We eat way too much salt, or sodium chloride. The sodium in the salt is what makes it harmful to the heart, blood vessels, and kidneys. We all know that too much salt causes high blood pressure. What we often don't realize is how much salt exists in food that we wouldn't even suspect. Remember when I said we need to cut through the clutter? Trying to figure out where salt resides in the foods we eat would test even Angela Lansbury as Jessica Fletcher's detective skills.

I know some of you add salt to your meals to give the food flavor. Some of you are probably even like my sister, who sprinkles salt on her food before she even tastes it. Instead, "taste before you shake." Remember, this is a learned behavior that you can change. There is no biological basis for this behavior. Salt is a habit, not a desire. It's something you learned and can unlearn.

People will often ask me if they should buy products with low sodium or reduced sodium. Most of the time, it's only about 25 percent less, which is still pretty high. I recommend to people that they use kosher salt, which usually has the least amount of sodium.

The real threat to your salt intake, however, is processed foods, and that's why I am so passionate that you need to reduce the amount of processed foods you eat. In fact, processed foods contain three-quarters of the sodium consumed by the average American per year.

Bread is the biggest culprit; it's the greatest source of sodium in the American diet. People get twice as much sodium from bread and rolls as they do from snacks such as potato chips, nachos, peanuts, and pretzels. Because pizza dough is typically made from white flour, pizza is a major source of excess salt. Other big sources are the processed meats I want you to avoid: lunch meats, cold cuts, and cured meats. I know many of you enjoy bacon, but there really are no health benefits to it. And don't think turkey bacon is a healthy alternative, because it isn't. It can actually have more sodium.

Americans consume an average of more than 3,300 milligrams of sodium a day. The American Heart Association states that sodium consumption should be less than 1,500 milligrams a day. So now you know another reason that processed food—especially white bread—has to go.

One tip I give people who have a lot of sodium in their diet is to eat a banana a day. Bananas are rich in potassium. Potassium can help the body to flush out excess sodium and might ultimately help you to become less addicted to salt. I also suggest that you replace salt with herbs and spices such as thyme, basil, rosemary, sage, chili powder, and parsley.

Diana Didn't Realize That Noodles Include a Lot of Sodium

Diana is a fifty-year-old woman who has struggled with high blood pressure for the past five years. She has also gained five pounds a year for the past three years, so when she came to me she was about fifteen pounds overweight.

"Dr. Whyte, no matter what I try, I can't stick with it," she said. "I get excited early on, but after a couple of weeks I lose enthusiasm." Diana has always been interested when I talk about dietary changes, and she seems very motivated and dives right into what I suggest. I think one of the problems is that she tries to take on too many changes all at once. Although Diana has not suffered a heart attack, her excess weight and high blood pressure put her at great risk.

At a recent visit, I decided that a new approach might be to tackle one issue at a time, and first on the list was salt. We talked about how the problem is not just the salt we add to our meals but also the sodium content in the processed foods we eat. Diana loves instant noodles. "I got hooked on them in college and have just been eating them ever since," she admitted. "I'm not even sure I really like them, but I eat them all the time." Instant noodles have an enormous amount of salt, and I gently suggested that Diana focus on eliminating instant noodles.

At her next visit three months later, she said happily, "I did it! I stopped eating instant noodles. I guess I knew they had a lot of salt, but I overlooked it because I was used to eating them."

It turned out that all of the salt had been causing Diana to hold water and gain weight. At her most recent visit, she had lost seven pounds, and her blood pressure was normal.

Read Food Labels

As you know, I don't want you to count calories. But I do want you to look at food labels. You don't need to spend a lot of time studying them, but you should learn how to read and decipher these labels.

These are general guidelines for what I'd like you to strive for. Even if you cannot remember these numbers, it's easy to make comparisons between different brands. For instance, you can compare two yogurts. Even if you cannot remember that there should be less than 12 grams of sugar per serving, you can compare two cartons—if one has 25 grams and the other has 14 grams of sugar, it's easy to decide which one to choose. My wife and I compare labels all the time, and so should you.

I also tell people to check the ingredients list. The shorter the list, the better. If there are a lot of words you can't pronounce, that's a bad sign. A little-known fact is that the ingredients are listed in order of their prevalence in the food. So the first couple of ingredients are mainly what the food is made of. This is important, especially when looking at items such as bread. Multigrain, 100 percent wheat, and whole wheat are not the same. You should look for 100 percent whole grain or 100 percent whole wheat in the ingredients list, and it should be the first grain noted.

Remember, we'll be decreasing your consumption of processed foods, which is where you'll find food labels. I still want you to be familiar with them and the general guidelines, but I also want you to focus on the big picture of which food groups to include and which foods to exclude.

The Meal Plans—Ready, Set, Go!

The AARP New American Diet meal plans are simple and include a 7-day, 14-day, and 30-day plan. I realize people often want and need specific directions in the beginning about what to eat, how much to eat, and when to eat. The meal plans for the next thirty days will get you started on a new dietary pattern for life.

There are a few things to keep in mind:

- You are likely to be eating differently from your family and friends in the next thirty days. Ideally, you will have gotten their support to help you achieve success. Maybe by your example you can introduce them to a healthier, delicious way of eating.

- Embrace the changes you are making. It is fun to try new foods, new flavors, and new ways of cooking. Remember, a positive attitude is important!

- As you cook, consider preparing several meals at once. That way, you save a lot of time. Most of the recipes in this book are for one or two servings, but you could make extra chicken at dinner and have it for lunch or in an omelet the next day. A salad, sandwich, or soup at lunch could also serve as a dinner option. I certainly do not expect or want you to be in the kitchen three times a day to prepare each meal. At the beginning, you probably will spend more time in the kitchen than you used to, but as you become more comfortable and knowledgeable about food choices, you'll automatically be making healthy choices, whether it's in the kitchen or outside the kitchen.

- Many of the foods you are used to eating are probably gone, if you've cleaned out your kitchen as I recommended earlier. Other foods will simply be prepared in a different way. You'll see that I deemphasize highly processed foods; there are mostly *real* foods, not processed ones, in these meal plans. That's probably going to be a big change for you. Your portions are also likely to be smaller, but you will be eating more often because I include two snacks. I know that for many of you it is going to be hard to eat five times a day; it's a new routine. So I'm happy if you can start with just one snack for a few days and then move up to two snacks by the end of the week. Snacking really does work in helping you to eat less food and thereby lose weight. Remember, snacking doesn't mean potato chips and M&Ms.

- Olive oil (especially extra-virgin) or canola oil is used frequently, but no butter, margarine, or cooking sprays. The way you prepare food is important; it'll take a couple of times until you're comfortable with all the grilling, baking, and sautéing, but they are skills worth learning.

- There are lots of fruits and vegetables—in fact, on every day and at nearly every meal. They have lots of bulk but few calories—a great combination for weight loss. The preparation might be different from what you've been used to; when I list vegetables, it doesn't mean vegetables smothered in cheese or covered with cream sauces or butter. It'll take some time for you to get used to these new and healthier tastes. There are a lot of salads that I think you'll enjoy. You'll soon see some of the biggest benefits if you make these important changes.

I have tried not to repeat meals too often so you will have a lot of variety. Feel free, however, to eat some of the same meals you enjoy over and over. Some people tend to eat the same thing all the time for breakfast or lunch and maybe even dinner out of habit. Repetition is fine, especially if it means you're eating healthy, nutrient-dense foods. For me, breakfast is whole-grain cereal and a banana. The key is to make a habit of eating healthy and nutritious foods, not the unhealthy ones that most people eat.

In the beginning I would like you to experiment with different foods. If after a couple of weeks you want to eat only one or two of the items in the meal plan each time for breakfast or lunch, that's okay.

Best of all, the recipes for each of the dishes in these meal plans are included in chapter 8.

Week 1: The 7-Day Plan

I mentioned earlier that the first two weeks are especially important. During this time you're establishing new behaviors and food
preferences while weaning yourself from your previously
unhealthy choices. I want you to follow the meal plans for these
two weeks very closely. Avoid meals prepared outside the home
during this time, since you have less control over the quality of the
ingredients and the preparation.

I don't list beverages at each meal. That's because for the first
two weeks, you may drink only water and coffee. I'm getting rid
of most of the liquid calories, and I want you to drink water
before every meal: at least one 8-ounce glass, preferably two
glasses. I also would like you to drink coffee at least for breakfast—but after you eat, not while eating. Your coffee can have
low-fat milk but no sugar. Avoid artificial sweeteners, especially
in these first seven days. There's no legitimate reason to put
cream or artificial creamers in your coffee. It's a learned taste,
and you will unlearn it.

Keep in mind that caffeine is an appetite suppressant. That's
why I don't want you to drink coffee before you eat—I want you
to eat a hearty and healthy breakfast. The appetite suppressant is
helpful later in the morning to make sure you don't go on a food
binge (especially for sugar) as you might have in the past.

The breakfast meals are full of good carbohydrates, mostly
from fruits and whole grains, along with complete sources of protein. There are also plenty of healthy fats. I have included cereal in
the meal plans since I know many of you are used to cereal, and it
is also pretty fast to prepare. When choosing cereal, be sure it has
less than 12 grams of sugar per serving and at least 8 grams of fiber
per serving. Eat these breakfasts as planned, and you will start
your day off right, feeling satisfied throughout the morning. The
midmorning snack will keep your insulin levels steady, preventing the spikes that drive hunger at lunch and cause overeating.

You'll see that I have included plain Greek yogurt several
times for breakfast as well as in some other meals. What's so

special about Greek yogurt? Is it really that different from regular American yogurt? Actually, it is. Greek yogurt uses a different type of bacteria to ferment the milk, thereby giving it a tart taste. There's also a different straining process, which removes a lot of sugar, salt, and excess water. The result is a thicker, creamier product that is higher in protein but lower in sugar and carbohydrates than American-style yogurt. It also contains probiotics, which help the digestive system as well as the immune system. Plain Greek yogurt is a type of superfood—you definitely should try it!

Day 1

Breakfast: Oatmeal with fruit and nuts; 1 apple
Snack #1: 1 Banana
Lunch: Grilled chicken salad; 1 orange
Snack #2: Handful of almonds
Dinner: Baked wild salmon with lemon and herbs; brown rice and broccoli

Day 2

Breakfast: High-fiber cereal; low-fat milk; ten berries
Snack #1: Low-fat cottage cheese
Lunch: Roast turkey sandwich with avocado and provolone cheese on whole-wheat bread; five strawberries
Snack #2: Handful of walnuts
Dinner: Shrimp with sautéed vegetables

Day 3

Breakfast: Lox on whole-wheat bagel with onion and tomato; 1 banana
Snack #1: Two handfuls of edamame
Lunch: Shrimp salad; 1 pear
Snack #2: Handful of raisins
Dinner: Baked lime chicken with couscous and green beans

Day 4

Breakfast: Mediterranean egg sandwich; five strawberries

Snack #1: Plain Greek yogurt with walnuts and blueberries (mix it yourself)

Lunch: Grilled chicken sandwich with lettuce, tomato, cucumber, and zucchini on rye bread with mustard; 1 kiwi

Snack #2: Handful of grapes

Dinner: Herb-rubbed beef tenderloin with sautéed asparagus

Day 5

Breakfast: All-natural peanut butter and banana on whole-wheat toast; quarter cantaloupe

Snack #1: Eight baby carrots and hummus

Lunch: New American Diet tuna salad sandwich on multigrain, rye, or whole-wheat bread with grape tomatoes

Snack #2: Two kiwis

Dinner: Pan-seared scallops with citrus salsa

Day 6

Breakfast: Blueberry-banana smoothie; whole-wheat toast with almond butter

Snack #1: Five celery sticks with all-natural peanut butter

Lunch: Minestrone soup; 1 apple

Snack #2: Small container of unsweetened applesauce

Dinner: Whole-wheat pasta with spinach and wild salmon

Day 7

Breakfast: Plain Greek yogurt with blueberries and walnuts; rye toast; half a cantaloupe

Snack #1: Handful of nuts (peanuts, almonds, pecans, or cashews)

Lunch: Cranberry-turkey sandwich on whole-wheat bread

Snack #2: 1 peach

Dinner: Shredded chicken tacos

Congratulations! You have completed week 1. Let's do a check-in. Go ahead and weigh yourself.

Date:

Weight:

BMI:

Waist circumference:

If you've been following the plan, you will start to see your body responding. Most of you have probably lost a couple of pounds at this point. For the first few weeks, you should expect to lose a couple of pounds every four or five days. In general, it takes a week or two before you notice any changes, but they will steadily appear.

Are you doing okay with the smaller portions? Portion control is important. You have to be careful that you are not eating too much at meals. Remember, I don't want you to count calories, but I do want you to manage your portions.

How is the snacking coming along? Snacking is a critical component of weight loss; I realize that for many of you it may seem counterintuitive, but trust me. Starving yourself between meals does not result in long-term weight loss; maintaining steady insulin and glucose levels does. I don't want you to get too hungry between meals—that works against your weight-loss plans. Why? You will be even hungrier at your next meal. Of course, do not use snacks to overeat; portion control is important here, too.

Week 2: The 14-Day Plan

Day 8

Breakfast: Whole-grain cereal with low-fat milk

Snack #1: Plain Greek yogurt with blueberries and walnuts

Lunch: Citrus-salmon salad

Snack #2: All-natural peanut butter on five whole-wheat crackers

Dinner: Shrimp with tomatoes, olives, and couscous

Day 9

Breakfast: Blueberry-banana smoothie; rye toast
Snack #1: Handful of nuts (walnuts, almonds, or pistachios)
Lunch: Grilled chicken breast; 1 orange
Snack #2: Five whole-wheat crackers and one ounce of cheese
Dinner: Lemon-pepper tilapia with roasted asparagus

Day 10

Breakfast: Black bean omelet; whole-wheat toast; one kiwi
Snack #1: Quarter ounce of dark chocolate
Lunch: New American Diet tuna salad sandwich on multigrain,
    rye, or whole-wheat bread; 1 apple
Snack #2: Handful of berries
Dinner: Herb-rubbed beef tenderloin with sautéed asparagus

Day 11

Breakfast: Oatmeal with fruit and nuts; five strawberries
Snack #1: Handful of raisins
Lunch: Greek salad with shrimp
Snack #2: Watermelon chunks with crumbled feta cheese and mint
Dinner: Chicken with Gorgonzola cheese and pears

Day 12

Breakfast: Plain Greek yogurt with 2 teaspoons sunflower seeds;
    1 banana
Snack #1: Low-fat cottage cheese
Lunch: Quesadilla; 1 apple
Snack #2: Handful of almonds
Dinner: Grilled salmon; string beans

Day 13

Breakfast: Two hard-boiled eggs; 2 pieces rye toast (no butter)
Snack #1: Handful of nuts

Lunch: Cranberry-turkey sandwich on whole-wheat bread
Snack #2: Six whole-wheat crackers with hummus
Dinner: Flatiron flank steak with tomato-cucumber salad

Day 14

Breakfast: Black bean burrito; 1 banana
Snack #1: Twelve baby carrots with hummus
Lunch: Strawberry salad with sunflower seeds
Snack #2: Two sticks of string cheese; 1 pear
Dinner: Whole-wheat pasta with shrimp

Wow. You are nearly halfway to thirty days!

How are you feeling? You should definitely feel different from how you did before you started. Let's do a check-in. Go ahead and weigh yourself.

Date:
Weight:
BMI:
Waist circumference:

If you've been following the diet as planned, you can expect to have lost five to ten pounds at this point. Some of you might have lost a lot more, some of you a little less. Remember, it's slow and steady that wins the race.

Have you lost your cravings yet for ice cream and candy? Are you no longer interested in the taste of soda? I bet the ample servings of fruit are satisfying any sweet tooth you might have.

How are you enjoying the dinners? They're designed to be rich in fiber so you will feel full yet eat less. The additional fiber should also be helping with your digestion.

Are you enjoying the fish? Eating fish doesn't promote fat storage, as eating meat typically does. Experiment with different ways of preparation.

Now is a good time to assess if you really are making all the changes to your eating patterns. I'm sure some of you have missed some days or some meals that the plan describes. Remember, that's okay and to be expected. Realistically, most people still have some improvements to make at this halfway point. The key is to keep moving forward and have more and more days that you follow the plan.

Week 3 of the 30-Day Plan

Day 15

Breakfast: Black bean burrito
Snack #1: 1 pear
Lunch: Almond-chicken salad; a handful of grapes
Snack #2: Two sticks of low-fat mozzarella string cheese
Dinner: Pork medallions with roasted baby carrots

Day 16

Breakfast: Two oatmeal raisin waffles; glass of skim milk; 1 banana
Snack #1: Handful of unsweetened cranberries
Lunch: Greek veggie burger; quinoa salad
Snack #2: Five whole-wheat crackers with all-natural peanut butter
Dinner: Citrus halibut with capers and diced tomatoes

Day 17

Breakfast: Whole-wheat French toast
Snack #1: Ten to fifteen grapes
Lunch: Black bean burrito; steamed kale
Snack #2: Watermelon chunks with crumbled feta cheese and mint
Dinner: Tangerine-ginger pork chops; steamed green beans

Day 18

Breakfast: Steak and eggs
Snack #1: Two handfuls of mixed berries

Lunch: Chicken and dill souvlaki (shish kebab) in whole-wheat pita; five carrot sticks

Snack #2: Quarter ounce of dark chocolate

Dinner: Grilled shrimp with brown rice; brussels sprouts

Day 19

Breakfast: Grilled vegetable omelet

Snack #1: Five celery sticks and hummus

Lunch: Capri-style (mozzarella and tomato) salad; five whole-wheat crackers or two pieces of whole-wheat toast

Snack #2: Handful of mixed nuts

Dinner: Grilled wild salmon with yogurt sauce and brown rice; steamed green beans

Day 20

Breakfast: Frittata with spinach and grilled chicken

Snack #1: Handful of mixed nuts

Lunch: New American Diet tuna salad sandwich on multigrain, rye, or whole-wheat bread; 1 apple

Snack #2: Two plums

Dinner: Black bean chili, salad

Day 21

Breakfast: Mediterranean egg sandwich on whole-wheat toast

Snack #1: Low-fat cottage cheese

Lunch: Grilled beef in whole-wheat pita

Snack #2: Two handfuls of edamame

Dinner: Roast chicken with carrots and celery

Let's do a check-in. Go ahead and weigh yourself.

Date:

Weight:

BMI:

Waist circumference:

At this point, your tastes should be changing. Instead of craving soda and junk food, you should be enjoying water, fruits, vegetables, and whole grains. You shouldn't have to be thinking so much about making healthy choices; they should have become more of a habit.

Many people will have lost about ten to fifteen pounds at this point. If you have lost that much or more, terrific! If not, assess what you've been doing well and where there is room for improvement. Are you taking too many cheat days? Are you using healthy cooking methods? Are you eating too late at night? Are your portions the right size? As I've said all along, the AARP New American Diet is about healthy living long-term. Even if you haven't experienced weight loss yet, if you're following the meal plans, you are reducing your risk of heart disease, cancer, diabetes, and possibly Alzheimer's.

Week 4 of the 30-Day Plan

Day 22

Breakfast: Two oatmeal raisin waffles; glass of skim milk
Snack #1: Two handfuls of edamame
Lunch: Mediterranean turkey sandwich; 1 tangerine (or orange)
Snack #2: Watermelon chunks with crumbled feta cheese and mint
Dinner: Steak fajitas

Day 23

Breakfast: High-fiber cereal with skim milk; 1 banana
Snack #1: Quarter ounce of dark chocolate
Lunch: New American Diet tuna salad sandwich on multigrain, rye, or whole-wheat bread
Snack #2: Two handfuls of grapes
Dinner: Chicken kebabs with tomato salad

Day 24

> *Breakfast:* Plain Greek yogurt with blueberries and walnuts; 1 mango
> *Snack #1:* Handful of nuts
> *Lunch:* Chicken-walnut salad with apples
> *Snack #2:* Two hard-boiled eggs
> *Dinner:* Mediterranean tuna with spinach leaves

Day 25

> *Breakfast:* Mediterranean egg sandwich on whole-wheat toast; 1 orange
> *Snack #1:* Two figs
> *Lunch:* Chickpea salad with tomatoes
> *Snack #2:* Five celery sticks with all-natural peanut butter
> *Dinner:* Chicken cutlets with stewed tomatoes

Day 26

> *Breakfast:* Peanut butter and banana on whole-wheat toast; handful of cherries
> *Snack #1:* Eight baby carrots and hummus
> *Lunch:* Shrimp salad; five whole-wheat crackers
> *Snack #2:* Handful of unsalted macadamia nuts
> *Dinner:* Pistachio-crusted chicken; sautéed snow peas

Day 27

> *Breakfast:* Strawberry-vanilla smoothie; whole-wheat toast
> *Snack #1:* Low-fat cottage cheese
> *Lunch:* Grilled chicken sandwich with lettuce, tomato, cucumber, and zucchini on rye bread with mustard; 1 pear
> *Snack #2:* Quarter ounce of dark chocolate
> *Dinner:* Grilled halibut with lime; cauliflower mash made with steamed cauliflower florets

Day 28

Breakfast: Whole-wheat English muffin with all-natural peanut
   butter; 1 banana
Snack #1: Handful of raisins
Lunch: Capri-style salad; two pieces of whole-wheat toast
Snack #2: Six whole-wheat crackers with hummus
Dinner: Chicken scaloppine with sautéed spinach

Time for a check-in. Go ahead and weigh yourself.
Date:
Weight:
BMI:
Waist circumference:

After the first month you should definitely be able to see the results. You most likely will be noticing the changes, perhaps by looser-fitting clothes. I bet people are even commenting on how good you look. Most important, how are you feeling? Do you feel sexy? Vibrant? More energetic? The promise of the book is not just to lose weight but also to feel better and live longer.

The new patterns of eating—smaller meals, five times a day—should seem natural to you by now. You probably don't feel as hungry as often, since the foods in the meal plan are more filling and satisfying.

Final Two Days of the 30-Day Plan

Day 29

Breakfast: Oatmeal with fruit and nuts
Snack #1: 1 apple
Lunch: Chicken-walnut salad
Snack #2: Two handfuls of berries
Dinner: Lemon-pepper tilapia with green beans

Day 30

Breakfast: High-fiber cereal with skim milk; one-half cantaloupe
Snack #1: Low-fat cottage cheese
Lunch: New American Diet tuna salad sandwich on multigrain,
    rye, or whole-wheat bread; handful of cherries
Snack #2: Two figs
Dinner: Whole-wheat pasta with spinach and wild king salmon

Congratulations! It's been thirty days. You did it! Let's do a check-in. Go ahead and weigh yourself.

Date:

Weight:

BMI:

Waist circumference:

How much weight have you lost? How about your waist circumference—have you lost a few inches?

At thirty days, most people who have followed the diet plan have lost ten to twenty pounds and at least an inch from their waistlines. Some have lost even more weight, especially if they were initially fifty pounds or more overweight. In addition, many people have much better control of their blood sugar, and some show improvements in their cholesterol by this point. So please go ahead and get your blood sugar and cholesterol checked.

Different people have different responses to the meal plan. Some people cannot make all of the changes to their way of eating in thirty days. They need more time. When that is the case, they often do not lose a large amount of weight initially. In this circumstance, I often tell these people to start again. Remember, it takes twenty-one days to change a habit and create a new one, and it takes thirteen times of eating something to develop new food tastes. So it's important to follow the meal plan and guidelines very closely. Remember, this is about lifelong habits, not a quick fix. If you follow the AARP New American Diet, the weight loss will come.

It's Not Just about Food

Eating healthily and losing weight helps tremendously in your desire to feel better, have more energy, think more clearly, be sexier, fight disease, and live longer. I wanted to stay focused on food for thirty days, but there are some other things you should know about that can help you to be healthy and live longer. Continue reading and find out.

Jackie Lost Fifteen Pounds in Thirty Days

Jackie is a forty-five-year-old mother of two who had never lost the weight she gained while pregnant. Ten years after the birth of her second child, she was five feet one and weighed nearly 150 pounds. Jackie had tried at least six different diets over the past decade. The more radical they were, the more she seemed to gravitate toward them.

"I once ate cantaloupe for every meal for a week. I lost five pounds at the end of the week, but once I drank some water, I gained it all back," she joked.

For years I tried to explain to her that successful weight loss is about healthy eating, not gimmicks or fads. About a year ago, I finally got her to try the AARP New American Diet. "Shouldn't I count calories?" was her initial response. I explained that calories count but that she doesn't need to count them.

"Good. I don't think I ever added them up right anyway," she retorted. "It seems like I'm eating a lot with all the snacking. You sure that's right? After all, shouldn't I be eating less food, not more?" I explained to Jackie why snacking is important and that she is eating more often, but not more food. She nodded hesitatingly, as though not completely convinced.

By the end of the second week, Jackie had lost a pound. I asked her if she had been following the meal plan. She said she had, but I know patients well enough to know that I often have to ask the same question in different ways to get an accurate answer. I asked about portion sizes.

"Seriously, Dr. Whyte, those portions are too small," she said. "I'm hungry after the meal, and I sometimes end up eating the snacks with breakfast and lunch." I gently explained to Jackie that that's not how the plan works. "Fine, I'll try again," she said. Since Jackie hadn't really been following the plan, I asked her to start again at the beginning. She was not happy about that, but she said that she would.

A week later Jackie called me to tell me she had put the diet "on hold" because she had to travel out of town. I gave her some tips on eating healthily while on the road, but she preferred to wait. "I want to do this right," she responded.

A month went by; then Jackie came in for a follow-up appointment. She had started the meal plans two weeks ago and had lost eight pounds. "I think I'm starting to understand this," she said. "I've even been drinking water, and the weight hasn't come back. I'm not going to lie—this is hard work. But I'm going to keep at it as best as I can." I told her that this was a great attitude.

Two weeks later, Jackie called me to tell me she had lost a total of fifteen pounds in the last thirty days. "And I feel great!" she said. I felt pretty great, too, hearing that.

8

AARP New American Diet Recipes

Cooking at home can be stressful for some people, especially when you're trying new foods. I've kept the recipes pretty simple. All of the ingredients should be familiar to you. At first I'd like you to follow the recipes pretty closely, but as the weeks go by, if you want to make some healthy modifications to a recipe, like adding more vegetables and whole grains, go for it!

Breakfast

• •

Oatmeal Raisin Waffles

SERVINGS: 2

¾ cup whole-wheat flour
¼ cup oatmeal

½ teaspoon baking powder
¼ teaspoon salt
½ cup raisins
1 egg
½ cup milk
1 teaspoon light olive oil

In a medium-size bowl, whisk together the flour, oatmeal, baking powder, salt, raisins, and egg. Slowly add the milk and continue to mix. Cover and set aside for 10 minutes.

Heat a waffle maker on medium heat. Brush the sides of the waffle maker with the olive oil. Place a quarter of the mixture onto the waffle maker. Be careful to evenly distribute the batter. Close the waffle maker. Cook for 4–5 minutes.

• •

Oatmeal with Fruit and Nuts
SERVINGS: 2

Oatmeal always reminds me of my early childhood. Back then, I really didn't like oatmeal that much. Now I love it. It's quick and easy to make. Adding nuts and berries gives it great flavor and increases the health benefits. It will keep you satisfied all morning. Give it a try, and you'll see what I mean.

2 cups water
½ cup fat-free milk
2 cups old-fashioned rolled oats
1 cup blueberries
¼ cup raisins
⅓ cup chopped walnuts
1 teaspoon flaxseed (optional)

Add the water and milk to a medium saucepan and bring to a boil. Stir in the oats and return to a boil.

Reduce the heat to medium. Cook about 5 minutes or until most of the liquid is absorbed. Stir frequently.

Remove from the heat. Mix in the fruit and nuts.

Spoon the mixture into bowls. Add the flaxseed, if desired.

• •

Mediterranean Egg Sandwich

SERVINGS: 1

Many of my friends enjoy egg sandwiches that are sold at fast-food restaurants. I think you'll find that this recipe is not only healthier than the Standard American Diet version—it's also much tastier. And the time it takes to prepare, cook, and clean up is probably faster than driving, waiting in line, paying, and then eating at a fast-food restaurant.

    2 teaspoons extra-virgin olive oil
    ½ green pepper, chopped
    1 egg
    1 egg white
    ½ teaspoon fresh oregano
    1 tablespoon crumbled feta cheese
    ¼ avocado, mashed
    2 slices whole-wheat toast
    2 slices tomato

Place the olive oil in a medium nonstick skillet (or use a skillet with a light layer of regular olive oil) and heat over high heat. Sauté the green pepper for 2 minutes.

Place the egg, egg white, and oregano in a medium bowl and whisk.

Add the mixture to the pan. Cook over medium heat for 1–2 minutes. Add the feta cheese and stir. Cook until thickened.

Spread the avocado onto the whole-wheat toast. Add the tomato and top with the egg mixture.

• •

Blueberry-Banana Smoothie

SERVINGS: 2

I was introduced to smoothies a few years ago at the gym. If you're someone who has trouble eating breakfast, this is a quick and easy way to consume the right amount of healthy calories. Smoothies can also be a great midmorning or midafternoon snack. The recipe here has a low amount of sugar yet is packed with protein.

  1 cup blueberries (frozen fruit is okay)
  1 banana
  2 cups skim milk
  2 tablespoons water or 1 cup ice cubes
  1 teaspoon vanilla extract

Place all of the ingredients in a blender. Blend until smooth.

• •

Strawberry-Vanilla Smoothie

SERVINGS: 2

I've added Greek yogurt as a twist to this traditional recipe, but I think you'll like it.

  1 5–6-ounce container vanilla Greek yogurt
  1 cup strawberries (frozen fruit is okay)
  1 cup skim milk
  3 ice cubes
  1 teaspoon flaxseed

Place all of the ingredients in a blender. Blend until smooth.

● ●

Peanut Butter and Banana on Whole-Wheat Toast

SERVINGS: 1

I know you might have grown up with peanut butter and jelly sandwiches, but once you try peanut butter and banana on whole-wheat toast, you'll be hooked.

1 tablespoon all-natural peanut butter

2 slices whole-wheat toast

1 medium-size banana, sliced

Spread the peanut butter on one piece of toast. Add the banana slices. Top with the second piece of toast.

● ●

Black Bean Omelet

SERVINGS: 2

The beauty of omelets is that they can be prepared so many different ways. A friend from medical school introduced me to this recipe years ago, and it remains one of my favorite breakfast meals.

2 large eggs

1 egg white

½ teaspoon freshly ground black pepper

¼ teaspoon kosher salt

2 teaspoons olive oil

¾ cup canned black beans (no salt added), rinsed and drained

¼ cup shredded low-fat sharp cheddar cheese

1 tablespoon chopped scallions

½ teaspoon minced garlic

1 tomato, diced

½ teaspoon cilantro

Combine the eggs, egg white, pepper, and salt in a medium bowl. Whisk until blended.

Place the olive oil in a skillet over medium heat (or use a nonstick skillet). Add the mixture and cook for about 3 minutes. Add the beans, cheese, scallions, and garlic.

Loosen the omelet with a spatula and fold in half. Cook an additional 2 minutes on low heat, covered. (The cheese should be melted.) Slide the omelet onto a plate. Add the diced tomato and cilantro on top.

• •

Vegetable Burrito
SERVINGS: 1

2 teaspoons extra-virgin olive oil

1 cup sliced mushrooms

1 tomato, chopped

½ cup chopped green or red pepper

2 tablespoons chopped onion

1 egg

1 egg white

1 whole-wheat tortilla

In a small skillet, heat the olive oil (or use a nonstick pan) and add the mushrooms, tomato, peppers, and onion. Cook over medium heat for approximately 3 minutes.

Add the egg and the egg white. Scramble for 3–4 minutes.

Place the mixture in the center of the tortilla. Fold the sides in and roll to close.

• •

Whole-Wheat French Toast
SERVINGS: 2

You don't have to give up all of the foods you enjoy. Sometimes you just have to make a few modifications. In this case, use whole-wheat bread and skip the syrup. This dish will still be tasty.

> 2 eggs
> ⅓ cup skim milk
> ½ teaspoon vanilla
> 3–4 pieces whole-wheat bread, cut diagonally
> 1 teaspoon light olive oil
> 2 cups chopped strawberries, plus a few whole ones
> 1 tablespoon grated fresh ginger

Place the eggs, milk, and vanilla in a small bowl and whisk together.

Dip the bread pieces into the mixture until evenly coated on each side. Let the excess run off.

Place a sauté pan over medium heat. (You can also use a griddle at 325 degrees.) Add the olive oil to the pan, and then when it's heated, add the battered bread to the pan. Cook 2–3 minutes on each side. The bread should be golden brown on both sides.

As a substitute for syrup, place the chopped strawberries and grated ginger in a small saucepan and simmer for 10 minutes.

Top the French toast with the mixture. Add the whole strawberries to the side of the plate.

• •

Grilled Vegetable Omelet
SERVINGS: 2

> 1 zucchini, sliced
> 1 yellow squash, sliced
> 1 red bell pepper, sliced
> 1 onion, diced
> 2 teaspoons extra-virgin olive oil, plus extra for coating
> 2 eggs

1 egg white

1 tablespoon skim milk

Coat the vegetables with some olive oil. Grill or broil for 4–5 minutes. Flip the pieces and grill or broil for an additional 2 minutes.

Place the eggs, egg white, and milk into a bowl and whisk.

Add the rest of the olive oil to a large skillet over medium heat, or use a nonstick pan.

Pour the egg mixture in the skillet. Cook 3–5 minutes. Add the grilled vegetables, fold the omelet, and. cook an additional minute on low heat, covered.

• •

Frittata with Spinach and Grilled Chicken

SERVINGS: 2

At first glance, this looks a bit complicated, but it isn't. It might take a couple of times to master it, but it's worth it. My wife taught me how to make frittatas, and they are a nice and different way to start the day.

1 tablespoon extra-virgin olive oil

3 eggs

1 egg white

2 tablespoons low-fat milk

¼ teaspoon kosher salt

1 teaspoon minced garlic

1 medium onion, chopped

¼ teaspoon freshly ground black pepper

1 8-ounce package spinach, stems trimmed

2 ounces goat cheese

5 thin slices grilled chicken

Place the olive oil in a medium skillet on medium-high heat.

Break the eggs into a bowl and add the egg white, milk, and salt. Beat the mixture and pour it into the skillet. Add the garlic, onion, and black pepper. Let the bottom solidify; push the edges and let the still-liquid egg run onto the bottom.

Add the spinach and goat cheese. Add the grilled chicken.

When the top is no longer runny, cover the skillet with a plate and turn it over so the egg is tossed onto the plate. Flip the egg onto its other side back into the skillet and cook an additional minute.

Lunch

• •

Grilled Chicken Salad

SERVINGS: 2

2 skinless cooked chicken breasts, chopped or sliced

¾ cup seedless red grapes

¼ cup pine nuts or walnuts

4 cups spinach, mesclun, or mixed greens

2 tablespoons balsamic vinegar

¼ cup extra-virgin olive oil

Put all of the ingredients in a large bowl. Toss well.

• •

Roast Turkey Sandwich with Avocado and Provolone Cheese

SERVINGS: 1

I'm not a big sandwich eater, since sandwiches too often consist of processed meat. But using carved fresh meat is a healthier way to still enjoy a sandwich. Be sure to try avocado, which gives it some extra taste and mouthfeel and provides the healthy fats your body needs. Provolone cheese provides a flavorful addition to the turkey.

4 slices fresh-cooked turkey

2 slices whole-wheat bread

½ cup mixed salad greens

¼ cup bean sprouts

4 slices avocado

1 slice provolone cheese

2 slices tomato

Arrange the turkey on one slice of bread. Pile on the salad greens, bean sprouts, avocado, cheese, and tomato. Top with the other slice of bread.

• •

Shrimp Salad
SERVINGS: 2

2 cups cooked shrimp

1 cup thinly sliced celery

½ cucumber, peeled and sliced

1 tablespoon lime or lemon juice

½ avocado, sliced

1 teaspoon flaxseed

mixed greens

In a medium bowl, mix together the shrimp, celery, cucumber, and lime or lemon juice. Add the avocado slices and flaxseed.

Serve over the greens.

• •

Grilled Chicken Sandwich
SERVINGS: 1

A grilled chicken sandwich is one of the healthiest meals you can prepare. You definitely need to give this recipe a try.

1 tablespoon Dijon mustard

2 slices rye bread (toasted, if desired)

1 skinless cooked chicken breast, cut in half

2 lettuce leaves

2 slices tomato

4 slices cucumber, peeled

4 slices zucchini

Spread the Dijon mustard on one side of each slice of bread. Place the chicken on one bread slice. Add the lettuce, tomato, cucumber, and zucchini. Top with the other slice of bread.

• •

New American Diet Tuna Salad Sandwich

SERVINGS: 1

This is my old standby. When we think about fast food, we should think about tuna fish. It's superquick, inexpensive, and very healthy. I try to eat it several times a month. Try this version—it's light and delicious.

1 6-ounce can light tuna fish, either water- or oil-packed, drained

¼ cup diced celery

½ onion, finely chopped

½ teaspoon lemon juice

chopped walnuts (optional)

1 slice tomato

2 lettuce leaves, sliced in half

1 or 2 slices multigrain, rye, or whole-wheat bread (toasted, if desired)

Mix the tuna, celery, onion, lemon juice, and walnuts in a bowl. Put the tomato and lettuce on the bread and add the tuna salad. Top with a second slice of bread, if desired.

• •

Minestrone Soup

SERVINGS: 2–3

My mother always used to make minestrone soup for us while I was growing up. Home-made soup is the best, and thanks to Mom, I'm able to provide this recipe with a few tweaks by me!

3 tablespoons extra-virgin olive oil
1 tablespoon minced garlic
1 cup chopped onion
1 cup chopped celery
1 cup chopped carrots
2 cups chopped tomato
1 can white beans
4 cups chicken stock
⅓ cup whole-wheat orzo pasta
1 cup chopped zucchini
1 cup baby spinach
½ teaspoon kosher salt

Place 2 tablespoons of the olive oil and the garlic in a medium sauté pan on medium heat. Add the onions, celery, and carrots and cook for 9–10 minutes. Add the tomatoes and white beans and cook for 4–5 minutes. Add the chicken stock, bring to a simmer, and cook for 20 minutes. Add the orzo and cook for 12–15 minutes.

Heat a sauté pan over high heat with the remaining tablespoon of olive oil. Add the zucchini and spinach and sauté for about 2 minutes. Add to the soup.

Add the salt and serve.

• •

Cranberry-Turkey Sandwich
SERVINGS: 1

2 cups chopped cooked turkey breast
½ cup dried cranberries
½ cup plain Greek yogurt
1 teaspoon grated fresh ginger
½ teaspoon kosher salt
2 slices whole-wheat bread
5–6 spinach leaves, stems trimmed

Combine the turkey, cranberries, yogurt, ginger, and salt in a medium bowl. Toss gently.

Top one slice of bread with spinach leaves, and then add the turkey mixture. Top with the other slice of bread to form a sandwich.

• •

Citrus-Salmon Salad
SERVINGS: 2

This is one of my favorite salads. We all know the health benefits of salmon; adding citrus gives it a punch of flavor and adds even more antioxidants. You won't find a salad that is much healthier than this one.

1 pink grapefruit
1 small orange (or tangerine)
1 tablespoon olive oil
½ red onion, thinly sliced
¼ teaspoon kosher salt
¼ teaspoon freshly ground black pepper
½ 8-ounce package spinach, stems trimmed
1 8-ounce salmon fillet, cooked
1 tablespoon sunflower seeds or ground flaxseed

Peel the grapefruit and orange. Over a bowl, separate the citrus sections. Save the juice in the bowl and put the citrus pieces aside. Add the olive oil, onion, salt, and pepper to the juice. Stir.

Add the fruit pieces and spinach to the bowl of juice. Toss gently.

Place the salad on a plate and top with the salmon. Sprinkle with the sunflower seeds or flaxseed.

• •

Greek Salad with Shrimp in Pita

SERVINGS: 2

My in-laws are Greek, and they love to include Greek salad at family gatherings. Recently, I've convinced them to "mix it up" a bit, and now they add boiled shrimp. They like it so much they've told their friends in Greece about it.

½ pound large shrimp, peeled and deveined

2 cups spinach leaves, stems trimmed

1 medium cucumber, peeled and sliced

2 medium tomatoes, cut into thin wedges

¼ cup kalamata olives

¼ cup chopped red onion

1 teaspoon lemon juice

1 teaspoon olive oil

¼ cup feta cheese

2 whole-wheat pita bread pockets, cut in half

Bring a medium pot of water to a boil. Add the shrimp and boil for approximately 5 minutes, until the shrimp turn pink. Drain and place the shrimp in a medium bowl.

In a large bowl, place the spinach, cucumber, tomatoes, olives, and onions. Toss, then add the shrimp. Add the lemon juice and olive oil and toss again. Add the feta cheese.

Serve inside the pita bread pockets.

• •

Quesadillas

SERVINGS: 2

2 ounces low-fat cream cheese

1 tomato, diced

2 8-inch whole-wheat tortillas

½ cup canned cannellini beans, rinsed and drained

¼ cup crumbled goat cheese

2 cups baby arugula

2 teaspoons olive oil

Put the cream cheese and tomatoes in a small bowl and stir. Spread the mixture evenly over each tortilla.

Using a fork, mash the beans and spread them over the cream cheese. Top with the goat cheese and arugula. Fold the tortillas in half.

Heat the olive oil in a large skillet over medium heat. Place the quesadillas in the pan and cook 2–3 minutes on each side, until the tortillas are golden and the cheese is melted.

Cut each quesadilla into 3 or 4 wedges.

• •

Strawberry Salad with Sunflower Seeds

SERVINGS: 1

My sister introduced me to this salad about two years ago. I never would have thought of a salad of strawberries, feta cheese, and mint, but I'm glad I learned about it. You will be, too! It's one of the tastiest salads you'll ever try, and it provides the variety that you need to keep your diet interesting and fun.

1 cup halved strawberries

2 teaspoons sunflower seeds

1 ounce crumbled goat cheese or feta cheese

¼ pound baby spinach or mixed greens

2 teaspoons raspberry vinegar

1 tablespoon extra-virgin olive oil

1 teaspoon chopped fresh mint (optional)

Place all of the ingredients in a medium bowl. Toss gently.

• •

Almond-Chicken Salad Sandwich

SERVINGS: 2

1½ tablespoons slivered almonds

1 4-ounce skinless cooked chicken breast, sliced

2 celery stalks, sliced

½ carton plain Greek yogurt

4 pieces rye or whole-wheat bread

Toast the almonds in a toaster oven or conventional oven, if desired. Transfer the almonds to a medium bowl and add the chicken, celery, and yogurt. Stir gently.

Place half of the mixture on one slice of bread and top with a second slice. Repeat with the other two slices of bread.

• •

Greek Veggie Burger with Quinoa Salad

SERVINGS: 4

For all the burger lovers, this is a twist I think you'll enjoy. At first glance, you might think, "It's only a veggie burger," but this recipe makes it quite tasty! It's even a little spicy. Give it a try—I bet you'll like it.

2 tablespoons extra-virgin olive oil

4 mushrooms, chopped

½ red bell pepper, chopped

1 carrot, grated

½ cup chopped spinach leaves, stems trimmed

2 tablespoons minced garlic

¼ teaspoon paprika

½ teaspoon cumin

½ teaspoon kosher salt

1 pinch cayenne pepper

1 16-ounce can chickpeas, rinsed and drained

1 10-ounce can black beans, rinsed and drained

½ 6-ounce can black olives

6 ounces rolled oats (and maybe some extra)

1 egg

1 tablespoon goat cheese

¼ cup sprouts

4 whole-grain buns (if desired)

Add 1 tablespoon of the olive oil to a large saucepan over medium heat. Add the mushrooms, red pepper, carrots, and spinach and sauté for 3–4 minutes. Add the garlic, paprika, cumin, salt, and cayenne pepper and cook for another minute.

Remove from heat. Add the chickpeas, black beans, and olives and mix thoroughly. Add the rolled oats and egg.

Form into 4 patties. If necessary, add more oats to hold the mixture together. Refrigerate for 30–60 minutes.

Add the remaining tablespoon of olive oil to a saucepan (or use a nonstick pan). Cook each patty 2–3 minutes on each side. Top with the cheese and sprouts. Serve on buns, if desired.

• •

Black Bean Burrito

SERVINGS: 2

2 whole-wheat tortillas

1½ tablespoons extra-virgin olive oil

1 onion, chopped

½ teaspoon minced garlic

½ yellow pepper, sliced

¼ teaspoon kosher salt

¼ teaspoon freshly ground black pepper

1 15–16 ounce can black beans, rinsed and drained

1 ounce low-fat cream cheese

1 tablespoon chopped fresh cilantro

Preheat the oven to 350 degrees. Bake the tortillas for 2–4 minutes.

Put the oil in a skillet over medium heat, sauté the onions and garlic, add the yellow pepper, and season with salt and pepper. Cook for 2 minutes, stirring occasionally.

Add the beans and cook for another 2–3 minutes, stirring a few times. Add the cream cheese and cook for 1 minute, making sure it melts. Add the cilantro.

Spoon half of the mixture into the center of each warm tortilla. Fold the sides in and roll the tortillas.

• •

Chicken and Dill Souvlaki in Whole-Wheat Pita

SERVINGS: 2

1½ tablespoons lemon juice

1½ tablespoons extra-virgin olive oil

¼ teaspoon kosher salt

¼ teaspoon freshly ground black pepper
½ cooked rotisserie chicken, sliced
1 cucumber, peeled and sliced
¼ cup sliced onion
1 tablespoon chopped fresh dill
2 whole-wheat pita bread pockets, cut in half
¼ cup plain Greek yogurt

In a bowl, combine the lemon juice, olive oil, salt, and pepper. Add the chicken, cucumbers, onions, and dill.

Fill the pita pockets with the chicken mixture and serve with a dollop of Greek yogurt on top.

• •

Capri-Style Salad
SERVINGS: 2

Tomatoes really are a superfood, so it's a good idea to know several recipes that include tomatoes. This one is a favorite. You might think of this as a summer dish, but it is one that can truly be enjoyed all year.

2 large tomatoes, thickly sliced
2 tablespoons extra-virgin olive oil
½ teaspoon freshly ground black pepper
5 ounces mozzarella cheese, thickly sliced
4 leaves fresh basil

Lay the tomato slices on a plate and sprinkle them with the olive oil and black pepper. Lay the slices of cheese over the tomatoes, and place the basil over the cheese.

Optional: Refrigerate, covered, for 45 minutes.

• •

Grilled Beef in Whole-Wheat Pita
SERVINGS: 2

My friend Judah, a personal trainer, gave me this recipe. He is always working to take unhealthy versions of food and make them healthy. This is a good example of using lean beef and combining it with some vegetables, a healthy fat, and whole grains.

  8 ounces cooked beef flank steak
  ¼ cup lime juice
  1 tablespoon chopped cilantro
  ¼ teaspoon kosher salt
  2 cups spinach leaves, stems trimmed, or mixed greens
  1 medium avocado, thinly sliced
  2 whole-wheat pita bread pockets, cut in half

Slice the cooked beef into strips against the grain.

Place the beef, lime juice, cilantro, salt, spinach or greens, and avocado into a bowl and mix well.

Fill each pita pocket.

• •

Mediterranean Turkey Sandwich
SERVINGS: 1

2 tablespoons hummus (see the recipe on page 143)
2 slices whole-wheat bread
4 lettuce leaves or 1 cup spinach leaves, stems trimmed
4 ounces sliced roast turkey breast
½ cup peeled cucumber slices
¼ cup sliced red bell pepper

Spread the hummus on each bread slice. Place the lettuce or spinach, turkey, cucumber, and red pepper on top of one slice. Place the other slice on top. Cut in half, if desired.

• •

Chicken-Walnut Salad with Apples
SERVINGS: 2

2 cups chopped cooked chicken breast (not lunch meat)
½ cup chopped walnuts

½ cup chopped apple

1 6-ounce package mixed salad greens

red wine vinaigrette salad dressing (see the next recipe)

Place all of the ingredients except the dressing in a large bowl and mix. Drizzle with the red wine vinaigrette salad dressing.

• •

Red Wine Vinaigrette Salad Dressing

SERVINGS: 2

½ cup red wine vinegar

½ cup extra-virgin olive oil

¼ cup lemon juice

1 teaspoon Dijon mustard

¼ teaspoon freshly ground black pepper

Place all of the ingredients in a medium-size jar. Tighten the lid and shake well. Alternatively, you can mix the ingredients in a blender.

• •

Chickpea Salad with Tomatoes

SERVINGS: 2

2 16-ounce cans chickpeas, rinsed and drained

2 cups cherry tomatoes

1 tablespoon chopped parsley

1 tablespoon chopped basil

2 tablespoons lemon juice

2 tablespoons extra-virgin olive oil

Combine all of the ingredients in a medium bowl. Mix thoroughly.

• •

Hummus

SERVINGS: 2

Homemade hummus is one of the easiest Mediterranean recipes to make. From start to finish, it takes about fifteen minutes. It's one of the healthiest dips and spreads, and this recipe so much tastier than the hummus bought in the store.

    1 16-ounce can chickpeas, half the liquid drained
    4 teaspoons lemon juice
    1 clove garlic, crushed
    ½ teaspoon kosher salt
    1 tablespoon tahini (sesame paste)
    1–2 tablespoons extra-virgin olive oil
    1 handful pine nuts (optional)

Place the chickpeas (with the remaining liquid), lemon juice, garlic, salt, and tahini in a blender or food processor. Blend for 1–2 minutes, until smooth.

Place in a serving bowl. Create a shallow well in the center of the hummus and pour the olive oil in the well. Add the pine nuts, if desired.

Dinner

• •

Chicken Cutlets with Stewed Tomatoes

This is a dish that my family has made for generations. My grandmother made these cutlets, my mother made them, and now I make them. The key for this recipe is to use Italian bread crumbs and to dip the cutlets twice.

SERVES: 2

4 boneless, skinless chicken breasts (about 6 ounces each)

2 eggs, beaten

2 cups Italian bread crumbs

2 to 4 tablespoons extra-virgin olive oil for frying

1 14–15 oz can stewed tomatoes

Place the chicken breasts on waxed paper or parchment paper.

Beat two eggs in a mixing bowl. Dip each chicken breast individually in the egg batter mixture. Place the chicken back onto the waxed paper.

Pour the bread crumbs onto the chicken breast on one side. Flip. Coat with the bread crumbs on the other side.

Dip each piece again in the egg mixture. Coat each side again with the bread crumbs.

Place a large skillet over medium-high heat. Add 2 tablespoons of the oil. Heat for 2 minutes. Add the cutlets to the pan. Fry each side for approximately 3 minutes. The chicken should be golden brown.

Place the chicken cutlets on a serving dish.

Pour the stewed tomatoes into a medium saucepan over medium heat. Heat for 4–5 minutes.

Spoon 1–2 tablespoons of the stewed tomatoes onto each cutlet.

• •

Baked Wild Salmon with Lemon and Herbs with Brown Rice and Broccoli

SERVINGS: 2

There are lots of different ways to cook salmon. This is one of my wife's and my favorites. The lemon and herbs as well as the brown rice (instead of white rice) provide a flavor that's hard to match. Add in the broccoli, and it will keep you full until the next morning.

Salmon
  1½ teaspoons chopped fresh dill
  1½ teaspoons chopped fresh thyme
  ¼ teaspoon kosher salt
  ¼ teaspoon freshly ground black pepper
  2 tablespoons extra-virgin olive oil
  2 6-ounce wild salmon fillets
  1 lemon, thinly sliced

Preheat the oven to 400 degrees.

Mix the dill, thyme, salt, and pepper in a bowl and set aside.

Add 1 tablespoon of the olive oil to a skillet or use a non-stick pan. Put the salmon fillets skin side down in the pan and rub the top of each fillet with the other tablespoon of olive oil.

Sprinkle the top of the fillets with the spice mixture. Lay the lemon slices on top of the fillets, completely covering the top of each fillet.

Bake for 15–20 minutes, until the salmon is cooked and becomes flaky when pierced with a fork.

Brown Rice
  See the brown rice recipe under "Side Dishes."

Broccoli
  See the broccoli recipe under "Side Dishes."

• •

Shrimp with Sautéed Vegetables
SERVINGS: 2

I will admit it. I love shrimp! This takes less than 15 minutes to make from start to finish. It provides healthy carbs, fat, and protein in the right amounts, all in one dish.

2 tablespoons olive oil

½ teaspoon minced garlic

½ medium onion, chopped

½ cup sugar snap peas

½ cup chopped broccoli

½ cup chopped cauliflower

½ cup baby carrots cut in half lengthwise

½ cup chopped red bell pepper

¾ pound large shrimp, peeled and deveined

¼ teaspoon kosher salt

¼ teaspoon freshly ground black pepper

Heat the olive oil in a large skillet over medium heat. Add the garlic and onion and cook for 1 minute. Add the peas, broccoli, cauliflower, carrots, and red pepper and cook for 4–5 minutes, until the vegetables are the desired tenderness.

Sprinkle the shrimp with the salt and pepper. Add the shrimp to the skillet and continue cooking until the shrimp are cooked through and pink—about 4 minutes.

• •

Baked Lime Chicken

SERVINGS: 2

¼ cup lime juice

¼ cup extra-virgin olive oil

1 teaspoon sugar

1 tablespoon chopped cilantro

2 chicken breasts

Combine the lime juice, olive oil, sugar, and cilantro in a bowl and whisk to make the marinade. Put the marinade in a large plastic ziplock bag and add the chicken breasts. Marinate in the refrigerator for a minimum of 2 hours or overnight.

Preheat the oven to 400 degrees. Bake the chicken breasts for 20–25 minutes in the oven, turning once. Turn oven to broil for 1–2 minutes, until the chicken is crispy on the outside.

Sauce (for chicken)
   ½ cup low-sodium chicken broth
   1½ tablespoons lime juice
   1 tablespoon water

In a small saucepan, bring the chicken broth to a boil. Add the lime juice and water and cook over medium heat for 1 minute.

Pour 1 teaspoon of the sauce onto each chicken breast and serve.

• •

Herb-Rubbed Beef Tenderloin with Sautéed Asparagus

SERVINGS: 2

2½ tablespoons chopped mixed herbs (thyme, rosemary, chives, parsley)
¼ teaspoon kosher salt
½ teaspoon freshly ground black pepper
1 teaspoon Dijon mustard
1 teaspoon minced garlic
1 tablespoon olive oil
2 4-ounce slices filet mignon

Preheat the oven to 425 degrees.

In a small bowl, mix the herbs, salt, pepper, mustard, and garlic. Coat the steaks on both sides with the herb mixture.

Add the olive oil to a skillet on medium-high heat. When the oil is hot, sear the steaks on each side (about 2 minutes per side), until a crust forms.

Remove the steaks from the skillet and put into a non-stick baking dish. Bake for 20–25 minutes.

If you prefer your steaks medium rare or well done, cook for a shorter or longer period of time until it reaches your desired level of doneness.

Sautéed Asparagus
See the sautéed asparagus recipe under "Side Dishes."

• •

Pan-Seared Scallops with Citrus Salsa
SERVINGS: 2

The citrus salsa gives a nice tangy taste to the scallops. I discovered this dish from a friend two years ago during the summer. But I make it all year long!

1 pink grapefruit
1 orange
¾ cup diced avocado
¼ cup diced red onion
1 clove garlic, chopped
1½ tablespoons chopped cilantro
2 tablespoons freshly squeezed lime juice
¼ teaspoon kosher salt
1 tablespoon extra-virgin olive oil
1 pound large sea scallops (8)
½ teaspoon freshly ground black pepper

Peel the grapefruit and orange. Separate the segments and place them in a medium-size bowl. Add the avocado, onion, garlic, cilantro, lime juice, and salt. Toss and set aside.

Heat the olive oil in a large skillet (or use a nonstick pan) over medium-high heat. Season the scallops with the black pepper. Cook approximately 2½ minutes per side.

Transfer the scallops in equal portions onto two plates. Spoon the salsa over each scallop and around each plate.

Whole-Wheat Pasta with Spinach and Wild Salmon

SERVINGS: 2

½ box whole-wheat penne (or spaghetti)

1 clove garlic, minced

4 tablespoons extra-virgin olive oil

¼ cup chopped basil leaves

2 tablespoons capers

1 tablespoon lemon juice

1½ cups baby spinach

½ teaspoon kosher salt

2 4-ounce wild salmon fillets (available frozen nationwide)

1 tablespoon grated Parmesan cheese

Bring a large pot of water to a boil. Add the pasta and cook until al dente, about 10 minutes.

Drain the pasta and transfer to a large bowl. Add the garlic, 2 tablespoons of the olive oil, and the basil, capers, lemon juice, spinach, and salt. Toss.

Add the other 2 tablespoons of olive oil to a skillet on medium-high heat. Add the salmon and cook for approximately 3 minutes per side. Remove the salmon from the pan.

Add the salmon to the pasta. Sprinkle with the Parmesan cheese.

Shredded Chicken Tacos

SERVINGS: 2

Instead of the typical tacos that are made with corn tortillas and lots of red meat, I've modified this recipe to include healthy alternatives such as whole-wheat tortillas and chicken. It will be healthier—and tastier.

2 whole-wheat tortillas

½ pint grape tomatoes, cut in half

1 avocado, diced

1 green pepper, sliced

¼ cup diced red onion

¼ teaspoon kosher salt

2 cups shredded skinless cooked chicken breast

2 lime wedges

Heat the tortillas.

Mix the tomatoes, avocado, green pepper, red onion, and salt in a bowl.

Divide the chicken evenly among the tortillas. Top each with the avocado and tomato mix. Add the lime wedges on the side (to squeeze to taste).

• •

Shrimp with Tomatoes, Olives, and Couscous

SERVINGS: 2

Olives are a terrific source of antioxidants. I have tried to add olives into the recipes in several places and a work colleague suggested it as part of a shrimp dish. This is a recipe that you might not think of at first to include olives, but once you add them to it, you will understand why. Olives give added flavor.

1 tablespoon extra-virgin olive oil

1 onion, chopped

1 16-ounce can diced tomatoes

½ cup halved black olives

¼ teaspoon kosher salt

¼ teaspoon freshly ground black pepper

½ pound large shrimp, peeled and deveined

couscous (see the recipe under "Side Dishes")

Add the olive oil to a large saucepan on medium heat. Sauté the onions for 3–4 minutes. Add the tomatoes, olives, salt, and pepper. Simmer for 4–5 minutes, stirring occasionally.

Add the shrimp, cover the saucepan, and cook 3–4 minutes.

Serve with couscous.

• •

Lemon-Pepper Tilapia with Roasted Asparagus

SERVINGS: 2

When my friends think of fish, they don't often think of tilapia, but they should. It is delicious, easy to make, and has healthy fats.

    1 tablespoon extra-virgin olive oil
    1 tablespoon finely chopped shallot
    2 6-ounce tilapia fillets
    ½ teaspoon freshly ground black pepper
    ¼ teaspoon kosher salt
    ½ teaspoon parsley
    2 tablespoons lemon juice
    4 lemon wedges
    roasted asparagus (see the recipe under "Side Dishes")

Add the olive oil to a skillet on medium-high heat (or use a nonstick pan). When it's hot, add the shallots and cook for 1 minute until the shallots soften.

Sprinkle both sides of the fish with the pepper, salt, and parsley. Cook the fish for 2–3 minutes on each side, until the fish is flaky.

Sprinkle the lemon juice on top of the fish. Garnish with the lemon wedges and serve with roasted asparagus.

• •

Chicken with Gorgonzola Cheese and Pears

SERVINGS: 2

2 4-ounce skinless chicken breasts

¼ teaspoon paprika

¼ teaspoon kosher salt

¼ teaspoon freshly ground black pepper

1 teaspoon olive oil, divided

1 cup diced onion

1 pear, sliced

¼ cup Gorgonzola (or, if not available, blue) cheese

Season the chicken evenly with the paprika, salt, and pepper.

Add ½ teaspoon of the olive oil to a large skillet over medium-high heat. Add the chicken and cook 2–3 minutes on each side. Transfer the chicken to another dish, and cover with aluminum foil to keep warm.

Add the remaining ½ teaspoon of olive oil to the pan. Sauté the onions for 2 minutes.

Return the chicken to the skillet and cook for approximately 3 minutes. Add the pears. Sprinkle with the cheese and let it melt.

• •

Grilled Wild Salmon with Yogurt Sauce and Brown Rice

SERVINGS: 2

Wild salmon is one of the healthiest fish choices you can make, so it is important to incorporate salmon into your diet. Try to stay away from farmed salmon, which is more controversial. I have provided a few different preparations of wild salmon in this book, and this recipe, courtesy of my sister, Jackie, is one of my favorites.

1 cup plain Greek yogurt

½ cucumber, peeled and diced

¼ teaspoon kosher salt

¼ teaspoon freshly ground black pepper

½ teaspoon minced garlic

½ cup chopped fresh dill

1 tablespoon extra-virgin olive oil

2 6-ounce wild salmon fillets (available frozen nationwide)

brown rice (see recipe under "Side Dishes")

Place the yogurt into a medium-size bowl and add the cucumber, salt, pepper, garlic, and dill. Mix thoroughly.

Preheat the grill to high and brush it with oil. Brush both sides of the salmon fillets with oil and place them flesh side down on the grill. Cook 4–5 minutes on each side, turning once. The salmon should flake easily with a fork when done. Top with the yogurt sauce.

• •

Flatiron Flank Steak with Tomato-Cucumber Salad

SERVINGS: 2

I love cucumbers, and any chance I can add them to a recipe, I take it! I think they work well in this recipe. It's a fresh taste that complements the tomato as well as the steak.

1 teaspoon extra-virgin olive oil

1 12-ounce flank steak

¼ teaspoon kosher salt

¼ teaspoon freshly ground black pepper

Heat the oil in a stainless steel pan on medium high. When the pan is very hot, season the steak with the salt and pepper and add it to the pan. Cook the steak for 4–5 minutes on each side (it should be slightly firm).

Remove and place on cutting board. Let it rest for 5 minutes so the juices settle in the meat. Slice the steak thinly against the grain.

Tomato-Cucumber Salad
See the tomato-cucumber salad recipe under "Side Dishes."

• •

Whole-Wheat Pasta with Shrimp
SERVINGS: 2

½ box whole-wheat penne

8 ounces medium shrimp, peeled and deveined

1 jar marinara sauce

Bring a medium pot of water to a boil. Add the pasta and cook for 9–11 minutes, until al dente.

Bring another medium pot of water to a boil. Add the shrimp and boil for 3–4 minutes.

Place the marinara sauce in a medium-size saucepan. Add the cooked shrimp to the sauce and simmer for 4–5 minutes. Drain the pasta and add the shrimp sauce to it.

• •

Pork Medallions with Roasted Baby Carrots
SERVINGS: 2

This is one of my wife's favorite recipes. We don't eat too much meat, but we always find a few occasions during the year to make this recipe. We especially love the baby carrots.

2 tablespoons extra-virgin olive oil

1 teaspoon kosher salt

¼ teaspoon freshly ground black pepper

12 ounces pork tenderloin, cut into 6 slices

4–5 shallots

1 clove garlic, minced

½ cup sliced mushrooms

1 teaspoon chopped rosemary

½ teaspoon chopped sage

1 teaspoon chopped parsley

½ cup low-sodium chicken broth

roasted baby carrots (see the recipe under "Side Dishes")

Put 1 tablespoon of the olive oil in a medium-size skillet over medium-high heat.

Sprinkle the salt and pepper onto the pork medallions and brown them for 2 minutes on each side. Remove the pork from the pan and set aside.

In the same pan, heat the remaining tablespoon of olive oil on medium high. Add the shallots and garlic and cook for 1 minute. Add the mushrooms, rosemary, sage, and parsley. Cook for 5 minutes, until the mushrooms soften. Add the chicken broth and bring to a boil.

Turn the heat down to medium low, put the pork medallions back into the pan, and cover. Simmer for 10–15 minutes, until the pork is done throughout.

• •

Citrus Halibut with Capers and Diced Tomatoes

SERVINGS: 2

1½ teaspoons extra-virgin olive oil

1 clove garlic, minced

¼ cup orange juice

¼ cup chopped fresh parsley

1 tomato, diced

1 tablespoon capers

½ teaspoon kosher salt

½ teaspoon freshly ground black pepper

2 6-ounce halibut fillets

Heat 1 teaspoon of the olive oil in a large saucepan on medium high. Add the garlic and cook for about 30 seconds. Add the orange juice, parsley, diced tomatoes, and capers. Add ¼ teaspoon of the salt and ¼ teaspoon of the pepper and simmer over medium heat for 4 minutes.

Season the fish with the remaining ¼ teaspoon of salt and ¼ teaspoon of pepper.

Heat the remaining ½ teaspoon of olive oil in a skillet pan on medium high (or use a nonstick pan). Cook the fish for 4 minutes on each side, until the fish is opaque and done throughout.

Serve the fish with the caper and tomato mixture on top.

• •

Tangerine-Ginger Pork Chops
SERVINGS: 2

Ginger is a great flavor that we often overlook when preparing meals. One of my friends I still keep in touch with from high school suggested this recipe; it's a good recommendation.

2 tangerines

¼ teaspoon kosher salt

½ teaspoon freshly ground black pepper

½ teaspoon minced garlic

1½ teaspoons grated fresh ginger

2 4-ounce boneless center-cut pork loin chops (about ½-inch thick)

Squeeze the juice from the tangerines into a bowl. Add the salt, pepper, garlic, and ginger to the bowl. Add the pork chops to the bowl, coating both sides of each of them.

Using a nonstick skillet on medium heat, cook the pork chops for 4–5 minutes, turning once, until browned on both sides. Remove the pork chops from the pan.

Drizzle any remaining juice over the pork chops. Serve with green beans (see the recipe under "Side Dishes").

• •

Grilled Shrimp with Brown Rice

SERVINGS: 2

8 ounces large shrimp, peeled and deveined

1 small tomato, diced

1 tablespoon extra-virgin olive oil

1 teaspoon lemon juice

brown rice (see the recipe under "Side Dishes")

brussels sprouts (see the recipe under "Side Dishes")

Place the shrimp, tomato, olive oil, and lemon juice in a bowl and toss. Marinate for 30 minutes, if desired.

Grill or broil the shrimp for 3–4 minutes.

Serve with brown rice and roasted brussels sprouts.

• •

Black Bean Chili

SERVINGS: 2

½ onion, chopped

1 teaspoon minced garlic

1 cup cooked black beans (or 1 12-ounce can, rinsed and drained)

1½ cups diced tomatoes

1½ tablespoons chili powder

1 tablespoon chopped cilantro

Add the onion and garlic to a small pot of water and let stand for 5 minutes. Add the black beans, tomatoes, and chili powder. Cover and simmer on low heat for 20 minutes. Top with cilantro.

• •

Roast Chicken with Carrots and Celery
SERVINGS: 3–4

1 whole chicken

seasonings, including salt, pepper, oregano, rosemary, and parsley

15–20 baby carrots

6–8 stalks celery

Preheat the oven to 325 degrees.

Rinse the chicken with cold water and remove the giblets from inside. Lay the chicken, breast side up, in the sink and sprinkle the seasonings over it.

Place the chicken in a heavy roasting pan or large casserole dish, and arrange the carrots and celery alongside the meat. Bake for about 30 minutes per pound, until a meat thermometer reaches 160 degrees. Remove from the oven and serve.

• •

Steak Fajitas
SERVINGS: 2

1 8-ounce flank steak

1 small onion, diced

1 green pepper, sliced

1 teaspoon extra-virgin olive oil

1 teaspoon chopped fresh cilantro

½ teaspoon ground cumin

¼ teaspoon kosher salt

¼ teaspoon freshly ground black pepper

2 whole-wheat tortillas

1 tomato, diced

Cut the meat diagonally and across the grain into thin strips. Place in a large zip-top bag with the onion, pepper, oil, cilantro, cumin, salt, and pepper. Shake well.

Warm a large skillet over medium-high heat. Add the meat mixture. Cook for 5–6 minutes, stirring frequently.

Spoon the mixture onto the tortillas. Add the diced tomato.

• •

Mediterranean Tuna with Spinach Leaves
SERVINGS: 2

If you like tuna, you will especially like this preparation. The Dijon mustard and the capers along with the spinach leaves will make you feel as though you're dining on the Mediterranean Sea.

4 tablespoons extra-virgin olive oil, divided

2 4-ounce tuna steaks (½–¾ inches thick)

¼ teaspoon kosher salt

½ teaspoon freshly ground black pepper

1 tablespoon lemon juice

1 teaspoon Dijon mustard

1 package spinach leaves, stems trimmed, or mixed greens

1 tablespoon capers

Place 2 tablespoons of the olive oil in a grill pan over medium-high heat.

Season the tuna with the salt and pepper and add it to the pan. Cook for 2–3 minutes on each side. Cut the tuna lengthwise into several ¼-inch slices.

Combine the other 2 tablespoons of olive oil with the lemon juice and Dijon mustard in a medium bowl. Stir.

Place the spinach leaves or salad greens on a plate and top with the tuna steaks. Add the capers and drizzle the tuna with the dressing.

• •

Chicken Kebabs with Tomato Salad
SERVINGS: 2

2 skinless chicken breasts, cut into 2-inch pieces
2 teaspoons minced garlic
2 tablespoons extra-virgin olive oil
1 teaspoon fresh thyme
12 grape tomatoes, halved
1 scallion, chopped
1 tablespoon orange zest
4 6-inch skewers

Heat the grill to medium-high.

Place the chicken pieces, garlic, 1 tablespoon of the olive oil, and thyme into a bowl and mix.

Thread the chicken onto the skewers and place them on the grill. Cook for 8–10 minutes, turning them every few minutes.

In a bowl, mix the tomatoes, scallions, and orange zest with the remaining tablespoon of olive oil. Serve with the chicken.

• •

Pistachio-Crusted Chicken
SERVINGS: 2

You probably haven't thought of nuts and chicken in this type of preparation. The pistachios give a unique crunchy taste—it might even make you forget about fried chicken!

½ cup pistachios

2 egg whites

¼ teaspoon kosher salt

¼ teaspoon minced garlic

2 6-ounce skinless chicken breasts

Preheat the oven to 400 degrees.

Finely chop the pistachios in a food processor. Place the pistachio pieces and egg whites in a bowl and add the salt and garlic.

Dip the chicken pieces into the bowl, covering them with pistachios.

Put the chicken in a nonstick skillet over medium-high heat. Cook for 3–4 minutes on each side.

Place the pan in the oven uncovered and cook for approximately 15 minutes.

Serve with sautéed snow peas (see the recipe under "Side Dishes").

• •

Grilled Halibut with Lime and Cauliflower Mash

SERVINGS: 2

My wife and I have a special fondness for halibut, which was served at our wedding. The lime gives it a nice twist (pun intended).

2 6-ounce halibut fillets

2 tablespoons lime juice

¼ teaspoon kosher salt

½ teaspoon freshly ground black pepper

cauliflower mash (see the recipe under "Side Dishes")

Heat grill to medium high.

Brush 1 tablespoon of lime juice over each fillet. Add the salt and pepper.

Place the fillets on a nonstick grill rack. Grill for 3–4 minutes on each side.

• •

Chicken Scaloppine with Sautéed Spinach

SERVINGS: 2

2 tablespoons fresh lemon juice

½ teaspoon chopped fresh (or dried) sage

½ teaspoon kosher salt

¼ teaspoon freshly ground black pepper

1 egg

2 chicken breasts, pounded to ¼-inch thick cutlets

¼ cup Italian-style seasoned bread crumbs

2 tablespoons extra-virgin olive oil

½ clove garlic, minced

¼ cup low-sodium chicken broth

2 teaspoons capers

Combine the lemon juice, sage, salt, and pepper and brush the chicken cutlets with the mixture.

Beat the egg in a medium bowl. Pour the bread crumbs onto a plate. Dip the chicken cutlets in the egg first and then in the bread crumbs to cover both sides.

Heat the olive oil in a medium skillet on medium-high. When the oil is hot, add the chicken cutlets and cook them for 3–4 minutes on each side, until cooked through. Remove to a plate and cover to keep warm.

In the same pan, add the garlic and cook for 1 minute. Add the chicken broth and bring to a boil. Add the capers and cook for another minute.

Lay the chicken cutlets on top of the sautéed spinach on a plate. Pour the sauce over the chicken cutlets and serve.

Sautéed Spinach
See sautéed spinach recipe under "Side Dishes."

Side Dishes

• •

Roasted Asparagus
SERVINGS: 2

8–10 asparagus spears
1 teaspoon extra-virgin olive oil
¼ teaspoon kosher salt
¼ teaspoon freshly ground black pepper

Preheat the oven to 400 degrees.

Break off and discard the bottom third of each asparagus spear. Put the asparagus spears in a large bowl and drizzle with the olive oil. Add the salt and pepper. Mix it with your hands to ensure the asparagus is coated with the olive oil.

Place the asparagus in a shallow baking pan. Roast in the oven for 12–15 minutes, turning once.

• •

Tomato-Cucumber Salad
SERVINGS: 2

2 tomatoes, cut into wedges
1 cucumber, peeled and sliced ½-inch thick
1 teaspoon extra-virgin olive oil
¼ teaspoon oregano

Place tomatoes, cucumbers, and olive oil into a bowl. Sprinkle with the oregano and mix.

● ●

Roasted Baby Carrots and Rosemary

SERVINGS: 2

2 cups baby carrots cut in half lengthwise
⅛ cup extra-virgin olive oil
¼ cup chopped red onion
1 teaspoon rosemary
½ clove garlic, minced
½ teaspoon kosher salt
½ teaspoon freshly ground black pepper
⅛ cup lemon juice
1 teaspoon parsley

Preheat the oven to 400 degrees.

In a mixing bowl, toss the baby carrots with the olive oil to coat. Add the red onion, rosemary, garlic, salt, and pepper. Mix.

In a shallow baking pan, lay the carrots in a single layer and roast for 15 minutes, turning frequently, until the carrots are lightly browned. Once the carrots are finished, remove them from the oven. Sprinkle the lemon juice and parsley onto the carrots in a bowl and toss.

● ●

Sautéed Snow Peas

SERVINGS: 2

1 tablespoon olive oil
1 clove garlic
½ cup chopped onion
2 cups fresh snow peas
1 tablespoon lemon juice

In a large skillet, heat the olive oil on medium-high. Add the garlic and onion and cook for 2–3 minutes. Add the snow peas and lemon juice and cook for 3–4 minutes.

• •

Sautéed Spinach

SERVINGS: 2

2 tablespoons extra-virgin olive oil
1 clove garlic
¼ yellow onion, diced
5 cups fresh spinach, stems trimmed
1 tablespoon lemon juice
Pinch of kosher salt and freshly ground black pepper

In a very large skillet, heat the olive oil on medium high. Add the garlic and onions and cook for 3–4 minutes, until the onions soften. Add the spinach and cook for 2–3 minutes, tossing frequently, until the spinach wilts.

When the spinach is finished, drain it in a colander, put in a bowl, and sprinkle it with lemon juice, salt, and pepper.

• •

Cauliflower Mash

SERVINGS: 2

½ head cauliflower
¼ cup skim milk
¼ teaspoon kosher salt
pinch freshly ground black pepper
snipped chives (optional)

Break the cauliflower into chunks/florets.

In a medium saucepan filled with water, boil the cauliflower until tender (10–12 minutes). Remove the pan from the heat and drain all the water.

Add the milk, salt, and pepper. Mash the ingredients. Sprinkle a handful of chives on top, if desired.

• •

Roasted Kale

SERVINGS: 2

½ head kale

2 tablespoons extra-virgin olive oil

½ teaspoon minced garlic

¼ teaspoon kosher salt

¼ teaspoon freshly ground black pepper

Rinse the kale. Dry thoroughly and chop into bite-sized pieces. Place in a baking pan. Add the olive oil and garlic. Toss the kale leaves to make sure all are coated. Bake at 375 degrees for approximately 8 minutes or until crispy. The leaves should be lightly brown. Sprinkle with the salt and pepper and mix.

• •

Quinoa Salad

SERVINGS: 4

2 cups vegetable broth (or water)

1 cup quinoa

1 teaspoon minced garlic

2 tablespoons extra-virgin olive oil

1 teaspoon lemon juice

½ tomato, diced

¼ cup kalamata olives, sliced

1 teaspoon chopped parsley

¼ teaspoon kosher salt

⅛ cup feta cheese (crumbled)

In a medium saucepan, add the vegetable broth (or water). Add the quinoa and bring to a boil. Reduce to simmer and cover.

Cook the quinoa until tender, 12–15 minutes or until the water is absorbed.

Add the garlic, olive oil, lemon juice, tomato, olives, parsley, and salt. Toss gently. Add the feta cheese. Toss gently again and serve.

9

Reducing Your Risk of Disease: Cancer, Heart Disease, and Diabetes

We know for a fact from the NIH-AARP Study that obesity can shorten your life span and decrease the quality of your life. Research has determined that once your BMI is over 25 (overweight), there's a 31 percent increase in mortality for every five-point increase in BMI. The heavier you are, the greater your risk of dying is from all causes. But as I said earlier, the problem is not just dying; it's also about getting chronic diseases that prevent us from enjoying our lives as much as we could and should.

The most common conditions that are associated with excess weight are cancer, heart disease, and diabetes. More often than not, these can be prevented if you lose weight.

Diet and Cancer

There are very few words that strike fear in patients more than *cancer*. It's hard for physicians to tell their patients they have cancer, and it's extremely hard for the patients to hear they have cancer. Their immediate concern is that they're going to die—soon. Telling a patient that he or she has cancer is heart wrenching.

What is cancer, exactly? At the simplest level, cancer is a group of diseases characterized by abnormal cells that grow and spread uncontrollably. Cancer is caused by both genetics and the environment. You obviously cannot change who your parents are. But you can change certain aspects of your environment, such as sun exposure, tobacco use, obesity, poor nutrition, and physical inactivity. Environmental aspects that are harder for individuals to avoid are the pollutants and chemicals that exist in our air, our food, and our water supply. When we talk about fighting cancer, we need to talk not only about treatment but also about prevention. After all, isn't it better to never get a disease like cancer than to have to undergo a battle with it even if the treatment is successful?

I'm going to tell you something that many people have never heard before: being overweight increases your risk of getting cancer. That's right—those excess pounds can make you more prone to develop cancer of the breast, colon, endometrium (the lining of the uterus), kidney, esophagus, pancreas, gall bladder, thyroid, ovary, cervix, prostate, or brain, as well as multiple myeloma (bone marrow tumors) and Hodgkin's disease. Being overweight may also increase the recurrence of cancer in survivors of the disease and decrease the likelihood of survival with treatment. The American Cancer Society believes that one-third of all cancer deaths are due to poor nutrition and excess weight. That's right—one in three cancer deaths is most likely caused by what we eat and how much we eat as well as how active or inactive we are.

How can this be? It's probably not just because of the excess fat and the dangerous chemicals that fat can emit but also because of the copious amount of food additives that pervade much of our food supply. Some food additives are used to enhance taste; others are used strictly for appearance or to increase product shelf life. Like many other doctors, I am concerned that these additives might be doing more harm than good. The key to avoiding cancer-causing foods is recognizing which ingredients are carcinogens, or cancer promoters, and reading food labels to permanently avoid consuming foods with those ingredients. As I've already mentioned, this book is about giving you the power to control your weight and your health—and knowing what foods can increase your risk of cancer is part of that.

This does not mean you will definitely get cancer if you are overweight, nor does it even mean that if you already have cancer, it's always due to being overweight or eating certain foods. But since being overweight and eating certain foods do increase the risk, here are two things you need to do:

1. Eliminate extra pounds by eating healthy food and engaging in physical activity.

2. Choose the nutrient-dense foods that help to fight cancer. You don't want to shorten your life by eating foods that aren't healthy and actually cause disease. It's also not good enough to focus on what you exclude; what you include is equally important. Food can act as a helpful medicine, strengthening your body mentally and physically. You need to find these powerful foods. Food can also be a toxin, poisoning your body and making cells become cancerous. You need to avoid those foods and choose wisely.

How common is cancer? More than two million new cases are diagnosed each year. You might be surprised to learn that more men than women develop cancer. Approximately one in two men has a lifetime risk of developing cancer; for women it's one in three. Cancer is the second most common cause of death in the United States; heart disease is the first. Half a million people die of cancer each year. That translates to about fifteen hundred people a day.

The following tables from the American Cancer Society show the estimated new cases of cancer for 2012 in the United

States as well as the number of deaths that occur each year.

Estimated New Cancer Cases/Deaths in 2012

Men

 Prostate: 241/740

 Lung: 116/470

 Colorectal: 73/240

 Bladder: 55/600

 Skin: 44/250

 Kidney: 40/250

Women

 Breast: 226/870

 Lung: 109/690

 Colon: 70/040

 Uterine: 47/130

 Skin: 32/000

 Kidney: 24/520

 Ovarian: 22/280

Cancer Cases/Deaths Each Year

Men

 Lung: 87/750

 Prostate: 28/170

 Colon: 26/470

 Pancreatic: 18/850

 Kidney: 8/650

Women

 Lung: 72/590

 Breast: 39/510

 Colon: 25/220

 Ovarian: 15/500

 Brain: 5/980

I know it might be difficult to believe that our weight has an effect on whether we get cancer, but it does, and there is a wealth of data to support it. Let's go over some of the most pertinent facts.

Various scientific studies that compared obese patients to non-obese patients found that the obese patients had 5.4 times the rate of the non-obese for endometrial cancer, 3.6 times for gallbladder cancer, 2.4 times for cervical cancer, 1.7 times for colorectal cancer, 1.6 times for ovarian cancer, 1.5 times for breast cancer, and 1.3 times for prostate cancer. Those are just some of the examples. Let's look at a few of them more closely.

Breast Cancer

Breast cancer is the cancer that most women worry about; it is the second leading cause of cancer death for women after lung cancer. Today, approximately three million women are living with breast cancer—about two million have been diagnosed with the disease and an estimated one million do not yet know they have it. Close to forty thousand women died from breast cancer in 2012.

At the current rate, one in eight women will develop breast cancer. When we look at the effect of obesity on breast cancer in postmenopausal women, it's truly shocking. A postmenopausal woman doubles her risk for breast cancer if she had gained as little as twenty pounds before menopause (especially between the ages of eighteen and thirty-five).

Being overweight is not the only risk factor. Your risk also increases if you drink more than one glass of alcohol daily. The risk of breast cancer is increased with the quantity consumed: studies have shown that women who had two or more drinks per day had a rate of breast cancer approximately 1.5 times higher than women who never consumed alcohol. We are not sure exactly why that's the case, but we believe it's due to the direct effect of alcohol on breast tissue.

Some data show that a diet high in omega-3 fatty acids can reduce a person's risk of breast cancer. Preliminary data also show that broccoli and Swiss chard might have a protective effect through plant chemicals such as indole-3-carbinol and natural carotenoids. Coffee may also play a protective role: recent studies have shown that women who drank two cups of coffee a day had a lower incidence of breast cancer than those who drank little or no coffee daily.

Endometrial Cancer

Endometrial cancer is the most common type of uterine cancer; the endometrium is the lining of the uterus. Although the exact cause of endometrial cancer is unknown, an increased level of estrogen appears to play a major role. Most cases of endometrial cancer occur between the ages of sixty and seventy, but a few cases have occurred before age forty.

As with breast cancer, the risk for endometrial cancer among postmenopausal women also increases with weight gain, and being overweight significantly increases the chances that a woman will die from endometrial cancer. This may be because estrogen is stored in fat tissue—so the more fat tissue there is, the more estrogen there is.

We have learned in recent years that drinking coffee may be protective here as well. Researchers found that women who drank more than four cups of coffee daily had a 25 percent lower rate of endometrial cancer than women who drank less than one cup daily. Some data suggest that soy-based products may reduce the risk of endometrial cancer, but more study is necessary before I'm willing to suggest that you start consuming a lot of soy products.

Prostate Cancer

Prostate cancer is the cancer that most men worry about; it's the second leading cause of cancer death for men after lung cancer. At the current rate, one in six men will be diagnosed with prostate cancer during his lifetime, and the disease kills nearly thirty thousand men each year. Prostate cancer doesn't usually start until age sixty; diagnosis in men younger than forty is quite rare—it happens, but not often. With proper screening and a healthy diet, many men can probably protect themselves against prostate cancer.

In recent years, we have learned from study after study that eating red meat and processed meat is associated with an increased rate of prostate cancer. We don't know why conclusively, but most doctors and scientists believe that it is most likely a result of the saturated fat in red meat and the nitrites in processed meat.

Saturated fats and nitrites are harmful to our bodies, which is why you need to avoid foods that contain them.

We also know that if a man drinks several glasses of milk (more than three servings a day) or eats a lot of dairy products, he may slightly increase his risk of developing prostate cancer. I still want you to drink milk and consume dairy, since we know from numerous other studies that the overall benefits of dairy outweigh the potential risks. The key is to keep the amount of daily dairy consumption to less than three servings and to be sure that it is low-fat.

Alcohol is also linked to this type of cancer. Consuming more than two drinks of alcohol daily increases the risk of prostate cancer.

What helps to reduce the risk? We have known for a long time that diets high in lycopene protect the prostate. Studies have consistently shown that about 50 milligrams of lycopene daily can reduce the rate of prostate cancer by 35 percent. Tomatoes are a great source of lycopene. So are watermelon, pink grapefruit, red cabbage, and beets. Not only red fruits and vegetables have lycopene, however—carrots and asparagus are also good sources. A cup of tomato soup typically has 25 milligrams of lycopene.

Marinara sauce, which you can put on pasta or chicken, easily has at least 50 milligrams. So definitely choose marinara sauce rather than cream sauce for your whole-wheat pasta!

Eating a plant-based diet lowers the risk of developing prostate cancer. Researchers in Seattle determined that men who ate three or more servings a week of cruciferous vegetables (cabbage, cauliflower, brussels sprouts, and broccoli) lowered their odds of developing prostate cancer by more than 40 percent than men who didn't eat these vegetables. We believe that this benefit is a result of two phytochemicals—glucosinolates and isothiocyanates—that seem to neutralize cancer-causing substances.

I mentioned earlier how healthy a diet high in omega-3 fatty acids can be. Several studies have shown that men who eat one or two servings of fatty fish weekly have a 63 percent lower rate of developing prostate cancer. We know that omega-3 lowers inflammation, and that's what might be in play here. So eat salmon and tuna.

Although I frequently mention drinking water and coffee, I encourage men to consider drinking green tea to prevent prostate cancer. Researchers in Italy studied a group of men who were at a high risk of developing cancer. The research found that those who took three 200-milligram capsules of green tea daily for one year developed cancer at a 90 percent lower rate than the men who took a placebo. We still need to do more studies, but green tea does have powerful antioxidants, which makes it a beverage to consider drinking—without adding sugar, of course.

There have been some instances in cancer research when we thought that a certain food, vitamin, or mineral prevented cancer. And then after further study, we learned we were wrong. Two recent examples are selenium and vitamin E. We used to think that these two nutrients reduced prostate cancer, but we now know from more studies that this is not the case.

Colon Cancer

Colon (or colorectal) cancer is a disease for which the risk is directly related to age: the older you are, the higher your risk. Nearly 90 percent of the cases are diagnosed in adults over age fifty. So if you are over fifty, this should give you another reason to start paying attention to what you are putting into your body, and paying attention to your stool (you need to discuss with your doctor any changes or blood in your stool).

Cancer of the colon is the third most common cancer in both men and women and accounts for 9 percent of all cancer deaths. Within the past few years, we have seen a decline in the incidence of colon cancer, largely as a result of good screening. Remember when Katie Couric had a colonoscopy on the *Today* show? That went a long way in getting people to consider having the test. I noticed years ago that colonoscopy appointments have the highest no-show rates of any appointments I've seen. It always seems that the car broke down, the date was forgotten, or the patient's child got sick. After Ms. Couric had her colonoscopy on TV, I actually received calls from people asking to schedule one. I'm very grateful to her for raising awareness.

If we can prevent cancer in the first place, shouldn't we try to do that? Some of the strongest data in research on food and cancer point to red meat and processed meat as increasing the risk of colon cancer. Again, it's most likely due to nitrites and saturated fat. Heavy alcohol consumption as well as smoking have also been shown to increase the risk. It shouldn't come as a surprise that high alcohol consumption can be toxic to your body, and we all know that cigarettes contain numerous poisonous substances.

One of the best ways to reduce your risk of colon cancer is to increase how many whole grains you eat and how often. We know from the NIH-AARP Study and other studies that adding up to three servings of a whole grain daily can result in a 20 percent reduced rate of colon cancer, with men benefiting more than women.

Whole-grain foods decrease the risk of colon cancer through various mechanisms, including increasing stool bulk, diluting harmful substances, and decreasing the transit time of food in the colon, thereby minimizing the time of contact between cancer-promoting substances and the lining of the colon.

I bet we could reduce colon cancer significantly if we stopped eating foods made with refined grains and replaced them with foods made from whole grains. Yet I find that this is one of the hardest behaviors for many people to adopt. Fruits and vegetables have also been shown to decrease the rate of colon cancer, though not to the same degree as whole grains. Consumption of milk and calcium appears to decrease the rate of colon cancer, in contrast to prostate cancer. The regular use of nonsteroidal anti-inflammatory drugs such as aspirin as well as postmenopausal hormone therapy may also reduce the risk, but these can cause other problems, so you need to talk to your doctor first to find out if these have value for your individual situation.

Head and Neck Cancer

Squamous cancers of the head and neck are the sixth leading cause of cancer death, resulting in 350,000 deaths annually. The major causes are tobacco and alcohol use. So not smoking and limiting your alcohol consumption will certainly decrease your risk of head and neck cancer, just as with many other cancers.

Head and neck cancer is another good example of how consuming fruits and vegetables is associated with a reduced risk. This isn't surprising. We know from the NIH-AARP Study that fruits and vegetables are rich in substances that we believe fight cancer, including folate, flavonoids, carotenoids, plant sterols, and vitamin C. All seem to be particularly protective against head and neck cancer.

Kidney Cancer

Kidney cancer is fairly uncommon, but we do know the major risk factors: smoking, high blood pressure, and obesity. So if you lose weight, you will reduce your risk of kidney cancer.

We've also learned from kidney cancer research that it's not just what you eat that matters; it's also sometimes how you prepare your food. Certain cooking methods for meat may increase the risk. When meat is overcooked through panfrying or grilling, some compounds form that might increase the risk of cancer. These include polycyclic aromatic hydrocarbons and heterocyclic amines. This is another reason to reduce meat consumption. When you do cook meat, be sure not to overheat and overcook it. I also recommend that you do not eat the charred portions. They most likely have higher levels of potentially dangerous compounds, and they're usually not even tasty.

The NIH-AARP Study has shown that five servings of vegetables and fruit daily decreased the rate of kidney cancer by approximately 40 percent. In particular, root vegetables (carrots, radishes, beets, parsnips, celery, sweet potatoes or yams, and turnips) appeared to reduce the rate of kidney cancer by up to 50 percent.

Key Points in Reducing the Risk of Cancer

I know you're not a scientist or a doctor, and I promised at the start of this book to break information down for you so you don't have to read a lot of studies and get confused. So I'll tell you what I found from the NIH-AARP Study and a few other well-designed studies to be critical when you are trying to reduce the risk of cancer.

The primary thing is to reduce your weight if you are overweight or obese. With the knowledge about the relation between cancer and weight, you have another reason to start being healthier and smarter in the way you eat. To reduce your weight and reduce your risk for cancer, you need to do four things:

1. *Eat more fruits and vegetables.* You should be eating at least three servings of vegetables and at least two servings of fruit daily, because almost all of the studies that have been done on this have shown that fruits and vegetables decrease the rate of cancer.

2. *Reduce your consumption of processed meat and red meat.* Study after study has consistently shown that the more processed meat and red meat you eat, the greater your risk of cancer is. No study has ever shown that eating red meat reduces cancer. I know that many of you like red meat, and the AARP New American Diet is not about completely eliminating foods you like from your diet. Instead, try to reduce your red meat consumption from every day to two days a week. When you do eat red meat, you need to look for the leanest cuts.

3. *Consume no more than three servings of dairy a day.* I don't want you to eliminate milk or cheese; I want you to choose low-fat products and not consume them more than three times a day.

4. *Limit your alcohol intake.* This means no more than two drinks per day for men and one drink per day for women, no more than three days a week.

Diet and Heart Disease

Although we discussed cancer first, you are actually more likely to die from heart disease than from any other illness. Heart disease accounts for nearly one in every four deaths annually—nearly six hundred thousand people die of it every year. In addition, more than twenty-five million Americans currently have some type of heart disease.

Genetics plays a role in whether you get heart disease, and so does age—there's nothing you can do about either. There are, however, risk factors that you can do something about. These include inactivity, obesity, cigarette smoking, high blood pressure, diabetes, and high cholesterol. More than one-third of Americans have two or more of these risk factors by the age of forty-five. What you eat affects every one of these risk factors, except for smoking.

It doesn't take a lot of weight gain or loss to have a significant effect on your heart and blood vessels. A weight gain of twenty pounds in middle age doubles your risk of heart disease. A loss of ten pounds will often reduce blood pressure back to a normal range.

The Skinny on Cholesterol

Let's look at cholesterol. Cholesterol is a waxy, fatlike substance that your body needs to function properly. You might be surprised to learn that, since the media often incorrectly portray cholesterol as something you should not consume. That's wrong; you never want to eliminate it completely from your diet. But when you have too much in your blood, it can build up on the walls of your arteries, the blood vessels that transport blood away from the heart. This buildup, called plaque, can cause a heart attack or a stroke. If you have high cholesterol (over 240 mg/dL), you are at twice the risk for a heart attack as someone at a normal level. So let's make sure your blood cholesterol either stays at or gets to a normal level.

Cholesterol level is determined by both genetics and diet. About 25 percent of our cholesterol comes from what we eat. Cholesterol does not exist in most food groups; it comes only from animal products. That's why what you put in your mouth is so important. If you treat food as a medicine, you might not actually need to take a prescription medicine like a statin to lower your blood cholesterol.

To lower your cholesterol, eat a diet that is low in cholesterol. You need to replace most meat products with plant-based foods (whole grains, nuts, and beans) and eat more fruits and vegetables. Consumption of just one serving of beans per day can reduce your risk of a heart attack by nearly 40 percent. That might be worth some occasional gas!

Does Oatmeal Really Lower Cholesterol?

You might remember seeing some television commercials a few years ago that claimed that eating oatmeal would lower your cholesterol. Those ads were true—oatmeal and oat bran can lower cholesterol. Oats contain a type of soluble fiber known as beta-glucan, which is also found in barley. It lowers cholesterol by binding to bile acids and removing them from the body.

Eating oats will therefore help if you have high or borderline cholesterol. Be sure to check out the oatmeal in the meal plan. But remember, butter-laden oatmeal cookies don't count! Instant packaged oatmeal with added sugar, artificial ingredients, and/or preservatives doesn't count, either.

Eating Fish versus Taking Medication

Eating fish rich in omega-3 fatty acids will reduce your cholesterol level. The fat in fish is monounsaturated and polyunsaturated, which is good fat. So instead of popping prescription pills to lower cholesterol, try to eat more fish such as salmon, sardines, and tuna. Fish sticks don't count, however! Ideally, eat fish two or three times a week. That might just be enough to avoid medication. And even if it isn't, fish has numerous other health benefits. Cooking method is important as well—baking and broiling is preferred; deep-frying often erases the health benefits.

Are Eggs Okay?

One of the biggest myths about food and cholesterol concerns the consumption of eggs. Eggs do contain cholesterol, so many people are afraid to eat them (or at least the yolks), but, in fact, eggs have many health benefits. They are low in calories, high in unsaturated fat, and high in vitamins, minerals, and protein. As long as you don't eat more than four eggs a week, your cholesterol should be fine. There's no evidence that eating up to four eggs a week, with the yolks, increases your risk of a heart attack. Remember, what you include is as important as what you exclude in your diet. Excluding eggs and replacing them with big, sugary, buttery muffins, for instance, does not help your health or your weight.

The Effect of Sugary Soda on Your Heart

Throughout this book I have explained why you should avoid soda. Sugary drinks can increase your risk of heart disease by 20 percent. Yes, that morning or afternoon soda you enjoy may possibly increase your risk of a heart attack. Studies show that even one can of sugared soda a day can lead to that increased risk. A 12-ounce can of regular soda contains 10 teaspoons of sugar; a 20-ounce can has more than 16 teaspoons (more than five tablespoons!) of sugar. We've learned over the last few years that soda, especially when it contains high-fructose corn syrup, which it almost always does these days, increases inflammation in our blood vessels, as evidenced by an increase in C-reactive protein. This inflammation can eventually cause the plaque I described earlier. The best option when you're thirsty is to drink water.

Do you need more proof that you should just drink water to reduce the risk of heart disease? We also know that sugar-sweetened beverages, especially soda, elevate blood pressure. A study of more than 2,600 people found that those who drank the most sugar-sweetened beverages had higher blood pressure than those who drank the least. In fact, adding just one extra sugary drink per day was associated with an increase in systolic blood pressure (the top number) of 1.6 points. That may not seem like much, but every few points above normal increases your risk. And high blood pressure increases your chance of having a debilitating heart attack or stroke.

Red Meat and Heart Disease

Meat seems to be the biggest problem for the health of our hearts. Numerous well-designed studies have consistently shown that consumption of both processed meat and unprocessed red meat is associated with an increased rate of death from heart disease. A recent study showed through nearly thirty years of follow-up that each additional serving of red meat per day was associated with a 13 to 20 percent increased rate of dying from heart disease, with the highest rate attributed to the consumption of processed meats. It was estimated that 9.3 percent of the deaths in men and 7.6 percent of the deaths in women could have been prevented by consuming less than half a serving of red meat.

As I explained earlier, the danger is most likely from the saturated fat and nitrites; high sodium in meat is also an issue. High-temperature cooking methods may release some toxic substances that affect the heart, just as they affect the kidneys. I know there are a lot of diets that focus on meat, but the information I am giving you is from thirty years of study. All of the meat in those high-protein diets is simply not good for our hearts and blood vessels.

Alcohol: Does It Really Help the Heart?

How does alcohol affect your heart? It looks as though moderate consumption of certain alcoholic beverages—specifically red wine—may reduce the rate of death from heart disease. It's important to point out that if you have an issue with alcohol dependence or liver disease you must not drink alcoholic drinks at all. A 17 percent reduction in the rate of stroke in women has also been found. This is probably because of flavonoids and other antioxidants, such as the resveratrol from the grapes used in red wine production. These flavonoids and antioxidants could also be increasing good cholesterol and might even prevent clots.

Antioxidants protect us from free radicals, which harm our blood vessels. These benefits have been seen only with red wine and not with any other type of alcohol. It is important to note, however, that the American Heart Association does not recommend drinking alcohol, including red wine, as a way of reducing the chances of heart disease. The reason is that many people do not limit their alcohol consumption, and they end up consuming more alcohol than they should. Too much alcohol causes numerous health problems, including alcoholism and possibly an increase in the risk of cancer.

If you enjoy wine, I do think there can be some benefits from a moderate consumption of red wine. There are different definitions of *moderate*, but if you have one glass of wine with dinner three days a week, you should be able to reap the benefits without exposing yourself to all of the risks. Those with alcohol dependency issues need to abstain from all alcohol consumption, of course.

Indulge with Chocolate

If you like chocolate, by all means indulge in it—but only a small piece a day (about a quarter ounce), and it has to be dark chocolate (at least 70 percent cacao). Studies have shown that the antioxidants, including flavonoids and polyphenols, in dark chocolate may protect our arteries from getting clogged and thereby prevent heart attacks. They may also decrease our blood pressure. It's the bitterness of the dark chocolate that signifies the presence of the antioxidants.

I'm not talking about America's beloved milk chocolate, which is highly processed. This is what most American candy is made of. (So my favorite, Milk Duds, doesn't count!) Rather, when the chocolate is close to its natural state, cacao, it contains powerful chemicals that can protect your blood vessels as well as increase your pleasure. Some studies have shown that consuming dark chocolate on a regular basis decreased the rate of stroke in women by 20 percent. So if you enjoy dark chocolate, I encourage you to eat some in moderation. (I told you this diet would include foods you enjoy!)

Diet and Diabetes

Diabetes is quickly becoming an epidemic. I bet you know someone with diabetes. More than 8 percent of the population has it—that's twenty-six million people. What's particularly frightening about that number is that only nineteen million know they have it; the other seven million people have diabetes and don't even know it. Moreover, nearly seventy-nine million people have prediabetes—this means you don't have diabetes yet, but you are borderline and likely to develop it if you don't change what you eat and lose weight. Many people think that diabetes happens only when you're young, but they are wrong. In fact, more than 25 percent of all Americans older than sixty-five have gotten diabetes.

Diabetes can be deadly. In fact, diabetes is believed to be directly responsible for more than 230,000 deaths each year. Having diabetes puts you more at risk for heart disease, stroke, high blood pressure, blindness, kidney disease, and gangrene. In fact, diabetes is the leading cause of blindness and kidney failure, and is the reason for more than 60 percent of limb amputations (rather than a trauma like a car accident). Diabetes is serious, but the most common type can largely be prevented by eating the right foods and maintaining a healthy weight.

What exactly is diabetes? Sometimes people with diabetes will say, "I think I have a touch of sugar." That's not completely accurate. There are two types of diabetes. Type 1 occurs when your pancreas does not make enough insulin. This usually occurs in children; its occurrence in adults is quite rare. Type 2 occurs primarily in adults; it used to be called adult onset diabetes, but now we see it in children as well because of childhood obesity. It occurs when the cells of the body become resistant to insulin and don't respond properly to it. This resistance eventually causes more and more insulin to be released, and the body still doesn't respond. The blood sugar level can get dangerously elevated, and that starts to cause all of the problems we just mentioned.

The symptoms of diabetes can be noticeable though not always obvious. Remember them as the three Ps: polyuria, polydipsia, and polyphagia. In nonmedical language that means you urinate a lot, you're thirsty a lot, and you eat a lot. Most people with diabetes have at least one of these symptoms. The diagnosis is pretty simple and can be determined by a blood test.

One of the biggest myths about diabetes is that eating too much sugar causes it. Sugar itself does not cause diabetes. Eating a lot of sugar will cause you to gain weight, and being overweight does increase your risk of developing type 2 diabetes. But a diet high in calories, whether from sugar, protein, or fat, will lead to obesity, and obesity is likely to lead to type 2 diabetes. Nearly 90 percent of type 2 diabetes is caused by obesity.

Preventing Diabetes

Type 2 diabetes can largely be prevented by eating the right foods and the right amounts. And if you already have diabetes, you may be able to get better control and even reduce the number of medicines you need by losing weight and eating healthy foods. If you lost 10 percent of your weight, you could probably eliminate diabetes, if you already have it, or prevent it completely. For instance, if you weigh 250 pounds, if you lost 25 pounds, you most likely would not have (or get) diabetes. Losing weight will improve your blood sugar readings while also improving the quality of life in patients with diabetes or prediabetes. It provides more energy, more vitality, better moods, and even a more active sex life.

Cutting back on your consumption of sugar may sound easy, but actually it isn't. You need to be a detective. Sugar is found in a lot of foods you wouldn't expect. For instance, some salad dressings have as much sugar as a candy bar. Ketchup has loads of added sugar, and so do cream substitutes. My mother loves flavored creamers; you guessed it—loads of sugar. I bet the reason you like barbecue sauce is that it has a load of sugar—check the label. And the California sushi roll that's so tasty? Guess what?

The carbohydrates in the white rice and imitation crab make it equivalent to a sugar cube.

Don't be fooled by low-fat products, either. As I mentioned before, they are often loaded with sugar to add flavor. It's easy to just snatch those products off the shelf without looking at them more closely. That's why you need to cut through the clutter and figure out what foods really are healthy and which are not. For a long time I thought granola bars were healthy. After all, they contain fruits, oats, and nuts. The reality is that many granola bars have more than fifteen grams of sugar—the same amount as some candy bars. They stay chewy through added molasses and other sugars. I do not eat granola bars, and I discourage you from doing so as well.

Whether you already have diabetes or are trying to reduce your risk of getting it, it's important to choose complex carbohydrates rather than simple carbohydrates as part of what you eat daily. The complex ones have a lot of fiber and keep your blood sugar level pretty even, preventing insulin spikes. They'll also make you feel full longer.

I need to point out that even though white potatoes are technically a complex carbohydrate, they mostly act as a simple carbohydrate. I tell people who are concerned about diabetes that eating a baked potato is similar to eating candy in terms of how the body treats it. And if you add butter, sour cream, or cheese, the way many people do, it's even worse.

If you have diabetes or are worried about diabetes, don't think you can't eat fruit. Studies have consistently shown that people who eat a variety of fruits and vegetables have a lower rate of developing diabetes than people who don't. The body seems to treat sugar from natural sources differently from added white sugar in food products.

Go Nuts

Don't be afraid to go nuts! Eating good fats, especially the monounsaturated fatty acids that are in nuts, can improve glycemic control. Two ounces of nuts daily as a replacement for carbohydrate foods improves people's blood sugar. The macronutrient profile of nuts fits well with a low-carbohydrate, high–vegetable fat, high-protein diet. If anything, nuts appear to be well suited as part of a plan to avoid diabetes, to improve its control, or even to lose weight. Just don't eat too many of them!

Red Meat and Diabetes

I have talked about the dangers of red meat for cancer and heart disease, and it turns out that too much red meat can also increase the risk of diabetes. A recent study of health-care professionals showed that a daily serving of red meat (the size of a deck of cards) increased the rate of type 2 diabetes by nearly 20 percent. Processed meat, such as hot dogs and bacon—which I've been telling you to avoid—increased the risk of diabetes by more than 50 percent. As we discussed earlier, the danger probably mainly comes from the nitrites and the saturated fat; excess iron is also a possibility. All of these make our bodies more resistant to insulin, and therefore our blood sugar eventually goes haywire.

When managing or preventing diabetes, you don't want to completely eliminate carbs, protein, or fat. You need all three to function properly. You simply have to choose good ones and eat them in moderation. This will help you to maintain a healthy weight and give you the proper nutrients for a steady insulin release that keeps the blood sugar level normal.

Patty Has Prediabetes

Patty is a very chatty fifty-year-old patient the entire office staff looks forward to seeing. On numerous occasions, she has delighted us by bringing in a homemade pecan pie. Patty is in pretty good health; she goes to the gym a few days a week, comes in for all her screenings, watches her cholesterol, and even checks her blood pressure at home. Her only problem is her blood sugar; it doesn't quite meet the definition of diabetes, but it has been trending that way.

Patty doesn't have a family history of diabetes. "You think it's the pecan pies, Dr. Whyte?" she asked. "I sure hope not. It would be hard for me to give that up. It's a family recipe, you know."

I explained to Patty what causes diabetes. I told her that sugar—even all of the sugar in pecan pies—doesn't cause diabetes. It's related to unhealthy eating habits that can contribute to obesity.

At the time of that visit, Patty was about fifteen pounds overweight for her age. Her weight had fluctuated for the past two years; sometimes it was a little less, sometimes a little more, but generally she was overweight by about fifteen pounds.

"Shouldn't the time I spend at the gym help?" she wondered. I explained to her that that has probably kept her prediabetes from turning into actual diabetes. But she was still taking too many calories in and not putting enough out. I suggested that since she was already active, she should try to reduce how much food she eats and improve the quality of her food.

I discussed drinking more water, eating oatmeal for breakfast, snacking in between meals, and eating less at each meal. I suggested that she consume more fish and not shy away from low-fat dairy. "What about the pecan pies?" Patty asked. I told her that was fine as a special treat every now and then, but not every week.

When Patty returned two months later, she had lost ten pounds. "I wasn't sure your diet suggestions would work," she commented, "but after I lost a couple of pounds the first week, I figured you knew what you were talking about, so I kept at it. By the way, I left you a present at the front desk." It was a pecan pie, which the staff had already started to enjoy!

10

Eat Well, Get Fit, Sharpen Your Brain

How long do you want to live? Eighty years? Ninety? One hundred? Just long enough to see your grandchildren graduate from high school or college? The number, or the goal, varies for each of us personally, based on our health as well as what's happening in our lives. The average life expectancy today is around eighty-one years for men and eighty-six years for women. Many scientists think that the average human body has the capability to live at least ninety years, and today we even hear of people living beyond one hundred.

How long we live is determined by two major factors: genes and lifestyle. Most people do not realize that our genetic makeup plays a small role in determining how long we live; experts believe it is only around 20 percent. Lifestyle—including what we eat, how much we eat, when we eat, and whether we exercise—accounts for 80 percent.

Research has shown that the genes we've inherited may make us more prone to developing various diseases, but they do not automatically cause them. The predisposition may never matter unless we make poor lifestyle choices that start a chain of events that lead to the disease. I mentioned that I have patients who tell me they have the "fat gene," so there's nothing they can do about their weight. Even if there *were* a fat gene, it would not automatically make them fat. Their eating habits also determine whether they are overweight. Genetics loads the gun, but lifestyle will pull the trigger. Developing a disease based on our genes is not inevitable. You really can exert a lot of control over your life by eating the right foods in the right amounts and by exercising. This book gives you the knowledge and the power to take control.

Of course, you want a longer life that is filled with energy, vitality, and good health. No one wants to live long in a frail and weakened condition with a brain that doesn't function properly anymore. How do you maximize your chances of living a long, healthy life? There is a mountain of scientific data in the NIH-AARP Study, as well as other research, to guide us.

Follow the AARP New American Diet

Certainly you need to eat a healthy diet. That is the most important thing you can do. Without a healthy diet, not only will you be overweight, but you'll also be shortening your life span by developing diseases like heart disease, diabetes, and cancer. In cultures with diets that primarily feature plant-based foods—fruits, vegetables, whole grains, legumes, seeds, and nuts—people live longer and have fewer preventable diseases than people in cultures that eat a lot of processed foods and red meat. The AARP New American Diet has plant-based components as well as fish and low-fat dairy, since we know that these help to prolong a vital life.

We've talked about how food is medicine that affects every part of your body. By reading this book, you now know how much your choice of food affects your chances of succumbing to certain diseases and ultimately the length and quality of your life. Our brains shrink and become less nimble as we get older, but healthier eating, focused on the foods in the AARP New American Diet, can slow the process. Using the results from the NIH-AARP Study, I've shown you the path to making the healthy food choices to live a long and healthy life. That's both the premise and the promise of the book.

It is important that are you are able to maintain the healthy choices you've learned in reading this book. I mentioned how most diets fail long-term because they are based on gimmicks, fads, and denial. The weight loss you achieve in following the AARP New American Diet is meant to be for life. That's why I have avoided counting calories and percentages of carbs, fat, and protein, and that's why I've avoided demonizing an entire food group. The AARP New American Diet has taught you a new way to think about food. The changes you've made—eating whole grains instead of processed grains, complex carbohydrates instead of simple sugars, and more fish and less meat, as well as drinking water instead of sugary beverages—will become so natural that you won't even need to think about making these healthy choices. You'll do it automatically, and that's what will sustain your weight loss.

You will stumble along the way, and that's not only okay; it's to be expected. The key is that you continue to move forward and that the majority of your choices are healthy and nutritious ones. Believe me, it gets easier and easier to make healthy choices. And you now have the knowledge and the power to do so. You've stopped kidding yourself, you've cut through the clutter, and you've made real change.

Move in Order to Lose Weight

But I'm not finished in helping you to be more vital, have more energy, and think more clearly. Food is one of the most important components, but it's not the only factor. Up until now, I have not really discussed exercise. In people who are overweight, poor nutrition accounts for 70 percent of the problem; physical inactivity accounts for the remaining 30 percent. Exercise is certainly important and does have numerous health benefits in addition to weight loss. All of us should exercise even if we are at a normal weight. It can lower our cholesterol, blood sugar, and blood pressure. It can prevent or delay osteoporosis.

Exercise also improves mood and can eliminate depression. It can improve your sex life by increasing blood flow and energy level. Ever hear of the runner's high? Runners have reported a feeling while running as though they had taken a drug like marijuana—they feel at peace and relaxed. Some people think this explains why runners keep doing an activity that puts a lot of strain on the body. Scientists have recently studied this phenomenon, and through the use of PET scans they have shown that some runners do indeed experience an increase in production of endorphins—the feel-good brain chemicals. The good news is that you don't need to put on your running shoes if you don't like to run; endorphin release can occur with all forms of exercise, not just running, and this general relaxed feeling and sense of well-being is good for your body.

Weight loss is an important result of exercise. Eating a healthy diet without exercising almost always results in regaining the weight. Exercise combats your body's attempt to regain the weight. It also helps in the calorie equation, burning more calories to maintain weight loss.

I want you to lose weight, and you will if you follow the AARP New American Diet. I also want you to become fit. What you eat and how much you eat as well as how you exercise and how often are all important. Studies have shown that men who were physically fit in their forties and who maintained that fitness for a decade reduced their rate of death from all causes in that decade by 30 percent, compared to men who were couch potatoes at forty. We have seen similar results in women. Those are better results than we see from any type of pill.

If you've been following the meal plans, you've been losing weight. It's important to incorporate exercise into the routine since it tones the muscles. I didn't want you to have to change too many things at once, so we focused solely on eating the right foods at the right times in the right amounts.

Now that you are mastering that, it's an appropriate time to increase your physical activity. Without exercise, weight loss may cause flabbiness in the skin as fat is lost from the subcutaneous tissue. This might change the shape of your body in a way that you don't like. Body image issues are important, and I want to make sure you are happy with your changing shape. So tone up!

How Much Exercise Is Enough?

How much do you need to exercise to get some health benefits? I'll be happy if you can do thirty minutes a day three days a week. Studies have found that even fifteen minutes of exercise a day translated into a 10 percent lower rate of cancer death and a 14 percent lower rate of death from any cause (during the time of the study), and the people who exercised fifteen minutes a day lived an average of three years longer than the people who didn't exercise at all.

But you have to do some activity that makes you sweat a little—just walking the dog for ten minutes is not enough (unless, of course, the dog weighs more than you do and drags you down the sidewalk the way my dog used to do when I was growing up!). How intense should exercise be? As you get older, it should be roughly 50 to 70 percent of your maximum heart rate (MHR). You calculate your MHR by subtracting your age from 220. So if you are 60, your MHR is $220 - 60 = 160$. Then 50 to 70 percent of 160 is 80 to 112. There are many different types of heart monitoring devices you can use to make sure you are in an effective and safe range. I recommend that you get such a device as you get older, since it is difficult to measure your pulse.

Another simple measure of exercise intensity is the "talk test." If you're doing moderate-intensity exercise, you can talk but not sing. If you're doing vigorous exercise, you can say only a few words without pausing. That's too intense as we get older. Aim for being able to talk but not sing.

Many people will say to me, "I'm too old to exercise," "I've never been athletic," or "I don't like to sweat. It messes up my hair." It's never too late to start being physically active. Even if you haven't moved off the couch in years, if you start exercising three days a week now, you can still receive the health benefits I mentioned in as little as six months. Find an activity or exercise that you enjoy so it doesn't seem like a chore. (And forget about your hair. Better to live longer with messy hair than to die sooner with neat hair!)

One of the best and simplest exercises is push-ups. Push-ups are great because they are a type of resistance training, which builds our bones and makes us less likely to fall and suffer a fracture. I recommend that people work up to twenty push-ups every morning and twenty more every evening. Most people can eventually work up to this number, even in a modified form, and there's no fancy equipment required. You can do push-ups any-where, so it's hard to find a legitimate excuse not to do them. I've had plenty of patients who couldn't do even one push-up when they first started. It might have taken them two to three months, but almost all of them have been able to work up to twenty at a time.

How Much You Walk Affects How Long You'll Live

I see a lot of elderly patients in my practice, and sometimes people will ask me how many years I think they have left to live. I don't always need expensive CT or PET scans to give me a sense of how well people are doing. The ability to exercise is one of the best and most accurate predictors of longevity. I learn a lot about someone simply by watching how well and how fast he or she walks. Some research has shown that people who could not walk a quarter of a mile in five minutes had a 30 percent greater chance of dying within three years than people who could walk that fast (and without problems or assistance). I tell all of my patients that they should get into the habit of walking.

The simple act of walking may also improve memory as we get older. It seems that people who walk more throughout life have greater brain volume than those who walk less.

How much should you walk? If you walk about seven miles a week, you may be half as likely to develop dementia as those who don't walk at all. I bet you're thinking, "Dr. Whyte, seven miles sure seems like a lot!" Actually it isn't. There are approximately two thousand steps in one mile, and most active people average about two thousand steps a day. You can check how many steps you take by getting a pedometer, which you wear on your belt or waistband, and it counts the number of steps you take. If you average two thousand steps a day, seven days a week, I'll be happy.

Exercise Your Brain, Too

At the Discovery Channel, we often say that our goal is to "entertain your brain." You not only need to entertain your brain; you also need to exercise your brain. So when you think about exercise as a way to increase your life span and the quality of it, you need to exercise your body as well as your mind.

We exercise the brain by learning new skills. It's good when we use skills we already have, such as playing the piano or the guitar, doing photography, painting, or writing poetry. But the reality is that using skills we are already good at doesn't make us smarter. Instead, we need to take up a new demanding activity that requires our brain to work.

Ballroom dancing is an example of an activity that is physically demanding but that also requires you to learn steps and execute them properly. (Didn't Ginger Rogers do all the dance steps that Fred Astaire did, only backward and in high heels?) So is learning to play an instrument, or if you already play one, to learn—and memorize—new music.

Even better is learning a foreign language. Patients often dismiss this idea, but it's one of the best ways to keep your brain well oiled and functioning on all of its cylinders. It requires memorization, proper grammar, and higher-level cognitive functions. It's a terrific workout for the brain, especially when we are older. Doing crossword puzzles is also a good idea, especially if it's a new hobby. I tell people that they should try adding up the cost of the items in their grocery cart rather than just waiting until the cashier tells them the number.

These challenging activities boost the brain's processing power and strengthen our neurocircuitry. We don't think of the brain as a muscle, but we should. And like the biceps, the brain needs to be flexed a little. So go ahead and practice memorizing. We know that if you practice memorizing, it builds up the area of the brain responsible for memory and research suggests that it might delay or prevent dementia. Delaying and preventing dementia will help you to live a vital, high-quality life. You'll do this by eating healthily, exercising your body, and exercising your brain. It's a perfect trifecta.

Have you heard of the word *exergaming*? This is a term used for video games that involve exercise. These enhanced virtual reality games that incorporate physical activity can delay cognitive decline even more than traditional exercise does. It's a twofer—it works your brain and your body, with benefits for both. I bet your children or perhaps your grandchildren play these types of games. I encourage you to get in on the act or even buy your own. There's no age limit for these, and the technology is really quite simple.

Global Longevity

Through my various jobs in the past fifteen years, I have had the opportunity to travel to almost every continent around the world. It's been an eye-opening experience in so many ways. I've been amazed that there are a few regions of the world where people tend to live to one hundred. I believe that if we could adopt some of their behaviors, then perhaps we too could live that long.

The Japanese island of Okinawa has the distinction of having the highest global percentage of centenarians. A close second is the

Italian island of Sardinia, which is one of the few places where men live as long as women—including up to the age of one hundred. Although these two islands are thousands of miles apart, they share some striking similarities. The prevalence of obesity is quite low— the majority of residents are at their ideal body weight. This is probably a result of the fact that their daily caloric consumption is roughly 80 percent of what we consume in the United States.

The diet in Sardinia is classic Mediterranean, which is rich in fish, fruits, nuts, olive oil, and vegetables, with little meat. The diet in Okinawa tends to be high in fruits and vegetables, with fish emphasized over meat. The people in both places seem relaxed. Obviously, I don't know if that truly is the case, but the constant rushing around we do in this country seems to be absent there, and I bet that the lower stress leads to a longer, happier life. Genetics may play a role, but lifestyle—especially diet—is a bigger determinant of longevity.

Frank Isn't Happy about Forgetting Where He Parks

Frank is a fifty-five-year-old man who called the clinic's urgent line asking to see me right away. Since he had been a patient of mine for some time, I made room in my schedule.

"I'm really concerned, Dr. Whyte," he explained. "I was at the shopping mall yesterday, and I forgot where I parked the car. It took me nearly half an hour until I found it. I'm afraid I might be getting Alzheimer's. Is there anything I can do to stop it?"

Frank is a fairly healthy man who is quite active. He is married with three adult children. He works in sales and is very successful in his job. Frank has had high blood pressure for the past ten years, but it's under pretty good control with medication. His only other issue is seasonal allergies.

Frank's father died of Alzheimer's disease about six years ago after a long illness, so Frank is quite concerned about his memory and mental health. I can sympathize with Frank, since my own father died of Alzheimer's.

I reassured Frank that forgetting where you parked is not a big concern. "I'd be more concerned if you forgot what type of car you drove, or if you couldn't remember how to drive to the office today," I said. The reality is that any type of dementia, including Alzheimer's, is quite unusual before the age of sixty. There are warning signs, and I went over them with him. These include trouble remembering how to do things you've done many times before, trouble managing money, difficulty following directions, changes in grooming, and the repetition of nonsensical phrases. Frank didn't exhibit any of them.

Frank still pressed me on what he could do. "What about supplements? Is there any special food I should eat?" he asked. I talked to him about the importance of healthy and nutritious eating, including whole grains, nuts, vegetables, and low-fat dairy. I described to him some of the recent data on coffee, berries, and fish. He is already pretty active, so I didn't need to remind him about exercise.

I know I didn't calm all of Frank's fears about dementia, but the tips I offered him will not only help him to prevent or delay Alzheimer's, but they will also help him to live a long and healthy life.

AARP New American Diet 6 Tips to Living Long

By reading this book, you know the importance of eating healthily in living a long and vital life. I have a few other tips that can help you to live longer:

1. *Get a good night's sleep.* It is important that you sleep seven to nine hours a night. Just as the right amount of sleep is

necessary for losing weight, it's also necessary for living longer. Studies have found than people who slept seven to nine hours a night lived longer than those who slept less. It is a myth that as we get older we need less sleep. Our sleep needs do not change over time. Our sleep often becomes lighter as we age, which leads us to wake up more easily. It also might take longer to fall asleep as we get older, but seven to nine hours is still the goal.

2. *Have a purpose.* We all know or have heard of cancer patients who by sheer willpower have lived to see the birth of a grandchild or watch a daughter walk down the aisle as a bride. I'm a firm believer that the brain has a powerful effect on the body. Simply wanting to be alive can make a difference.

3. *Stay positive.* I mentioned a couple of times how important it is to be positive in your weight-loss quest. Being positive might also help you to live longer. Being optimistic and cheerful has multiple benefits. A recent study of nearly four thousand men and women ages fifty-two to seventy-nine found that those who saw the world through rose-colored glasses had a 35 percent lower rate of dying within the next five years than those with the lowest happiness levels. This was the case even for those individuals with serious chronic illnesses—they lived longer when they were happy.

4. *Embrace java.* I'm a big supporter of coffee—and for good reason. I've mentioned the health benefits of coffee throughout this book. According to the NIH-AARP Study, coffee drinkers were less likely to die from heart disease, respiratory disease, stroke, injuries and accidents, diabetes, and infections. Here's one more piece of research: people who drank three to five cups of coffee a day in their forties and fifties had a 65 percent lower rate of developing Alzheimer's than those who drank two cups a day. This was regular coffee, not the fancy lattes, cappuccinos, or mochas with added fats and sugars.

5. *Stay connected.* Social isolation hastens the onset of dementia. It's great that people are connected online through social media, and that has value. It's also important to have the old-fashioned connections that involve having people over to your house, going out to dinner with family and friends, and being part of people's lives. Connections cannot just be virtual. You might want to join or start a reading group, or volunteer in your community. That way, you can stay connected with other people and exercise your brain at the same time.

6. *Get screened.* Depending on your age and overall health, you may need to be screened regularly to prevent disease. This includes screening for cholesterol, depression, diabetes, high blood pressure, and cancer. The U.S. Preventive Services Task Force publishes guidelines on who should be screened for what and at what age. Visit http://www .preventiveservicestaskforce.org to help you and your doctor determine what screening tests you need.

It is my sincere hope that the AARP New American Diet will help you and your loved ones live a long, healthy, and vital life. Here's to good eating!

References

This diet is largely based on research by the National Institutes of Health and AARP, the NIH-AARP Diet and Health Study, which can be found at http://dietandhealth.cancer.gov, as well as the other references listed here.

3. AARP New American Diet Nutrition Basics

It is amazing to see how portion sizes have changed over the years and how they relate to obesity. The information in this chapter is based on data from Centers for Disease Control and Prevention (CDC) and the National Institutes of Health (NIH). The CDC has excellent information on changing portion sizes that is available at http://www.cdc.gov/healthyweight/healthy_eating/portion_size.html.

The challenges in estimating portion sizes are well documented. Nutrition experts at Penn State University demonstrated the impact of portion size on weight management: Ello-Martin, J. A., J. H. Ledikwe, and B. J. Rolls. "The Influence of Food Portion Size and Energy Density on Energy Intake: Implications for Weight Management." *American Journal of Clinical Nutrition* 82, no. 1 (July 2005): 236–241S.

Researchers at Johns Hopkins University also showed how our poor math skills and our insufficient understanding of health terms affect our weight. Huizinga, M. M., A. J. Carlisle, K. L. Cavanaugh, D. L. Davis, R. P. Gregory, D. G. Schlundt, and R. L. Rothman. "Literacy, Numeracy, and Portion-Size Estimation Skills." *American Journal of Preventive Medicine* 36, no. 4 (April 2009): 324–328.

Our low consumption of fruits and vegetables has been going on for years. The CDC publishes a report on our annual intake. The trends are noteworthy, and the details can be viewed in a recent report. The data in this chapter are based on the following report: Centers for Disease Control. "State-Specific Trends in Fruit and Vegetable Consumption among Adults—United States, 2000–2009." *Morbidity and Mortality Weekly Report* 59, no. 35 (September 2010): 1125–1130.

Much of the nutrition information in this chapter is supported by CDC data. The CDC puts out excellent resources on nutrition basics that can be found at http://www.cdc.gov/nutrition/everyone/basics/index.html.

The information on vitamins and minerals is based on recommendations by the Institute of Medicine, which has developed a set of nutrient reference values called *dietary reference intakes*. These serve as a guide for good nutrition and provide the scientific basis for the development of food guidelines in the United States. They are specified on the basis of age, sex, and life stage and cover more than forty nutrient substances.

The latest data on vitamin D and calcium discussed in this chapter are based on the new dietary reference intakes for calcium and vitamin D: National Research Council. *Front Matter: Dietary Reference Intakes for Calcium and Vitamin D.* Washington, DC: National Academies Press, 2011.

The most recent data regarding the risk of too much vitamin D can be found in Amer, M., and R. Qayyum. "Relation between Serum 25-Hydroxyvitamin D and C-Reactive Protein in Asymptomatic Adults." Continuous National Health and Nutrition Examination Survey, 2001 to 2006. *American Journal of Cardiology* 109, no. 2 (2012): 226–230.

The information relating to the risk of vitamin supplements can be found in Mursu, J., K. Robien, L. J. Harnack, K. Park, and D. R. Jacobs. "Dietary Supplements and Mortality Rate in Older Women: The Iowa Women's Health Study." *Archives of Internal Medicine* 171, no. 18 (2011): 1625.

4. You Don't Have to Be Overweight

The obesity epidemic is well known. The National Center for Health Statistics provides some of the best and most reliable data on being overweight and obese. The data in this chapter are based on the most complete and accurate data for adults at the time of publication: Flegal, K. M., M. D. Carroll, B. K. Kit, and C. L. Ogden. "Prevalence of Obesity and Trends in the Distribution of Body Mass Index among US Adults, 1999–2010." *Journal of the American Medical Association* 307, no. 5 (February 1, 2012): 491–497.

Data on overweight and obese children can be found in Ogden, C. L., M. D. Carroll, B. K. Kit, and K. M. Flegal. "Prevalence of Obesity and Trends in Body Mass Index among US Children and Adolescents, 1999–2010." *Journal of the American Medical Association* 307, no. 5 (February 1, 2012): 483–490.

The information on body mass index and mortality has been studied extensively. The information in this chapter is largely based on the following:

De Gonzalez, B. "Body-Mass Index and Mortality among 1.46 Million White Adults." *New England Journal of Medicine* 363, no. 23 (December 2, 2010): 2211–2219.

Whitlock, [fi]. "Body-Mass Index and Cause-Specific Mortality in 900,000 Adults: Collaborative Analyses of 57 Prospective Studies." *Lancet* 373, no. 9669 (March 28, 2009): 1083–1096.

Scientists have been able to carve out the data by age, and that is addressed in this chapter. Information from the following study served as a basis for the chapter discussion: Adams, K. F., A. Schatzkin, T. B. Harris, V. Kipnis, T. Mouw, R. Ballard-Barbash, A. Hollenbeck, and M. F. Leitzmann. "Overweight, Obesity, and Mortality in a Large Prospective Cohort of Persons 50 to 71 Years Old." *New England Journal of Medicine* 355, no. 8 (August 24, 2006): 763–778.

The discussion on waist circumference continues to evolve. Much of the information in this chapter was based on the following studies:

Jacobs, E. J., C. C. Newton, Y. Wang, A. V. Patel, M. L. McCullough, P. T. Campbell, M. J. Thun, and S. M. Gapstur. "Waist Circumference and All-Cause Mortality in a Large US Cohort." *Archives of Internal Medicine* 170, no. 15 (August 9, 2010): 1293–1301.

Paula, H. A., R. D. Ribeiro, L. E. Rosado, M. V. Abranches, and S. D. Franceschini. "Classic Anthropometric and Body Composition Indicators Can Predict Risk of Metabolic Syndrome in Elderly." *Annals of Nutrition and Metabolism* 60, no. 4 (June 1, 2012): 264–271.

For the discussion on BMI versus waist circumference, data were obtained from the following studies:

Freiberg, M. S., M. J. Pencina, R. B. D'Agostino, K. Lanier, P. W. Wilson, and R. S. Vasan. "BMI vs. Waist Circumference for Identifying Vascular Risk." *Obesity* 16, no. 2 (February 2008): 463–469.

Janssen, I., P. T. Katzmarzyk, and R. Ross. "Body Mass Index Is Inversely Related to Mortality in Older People after Adjustment for Waist

Circumference." *Journal of the American Geriatric Society* 53, no. 12 (December 2005): 2112–2118.

I mentioned the need to weigh oneself, especially weekly in the early part of the AARP New American Diet. This recommendation is based on the following studies:

Butryn, M. L., S. Phelan, J. O. Hill, and R. R. Wing. "Consistent Self-Monitoring of Weight: A Key Component of Successful Weight Loss Maintenance." *Obesity* 15, no. 12 (December 2007): 3091–3096.

VanWormer, J. J., S. A. French, M. A. Pereira, and E. M. Welsh. "The Impact of Regular Self-Weighing on Weight Management: A Systematic Literature Review." *International Journal of Behavioral Nutrition and Physical Activity* 5 (November 4, 2008): 54.

VanWormer, J. J., A. M. Martinez, B. C. Martinson, A. L. Crain, G. A. Benson, D. L. Cosentino, and N. P. Pronk. "Self-Weighing Promotes Weight Loss for Obese Adults." *American Journal of Preventive Medicine* 36, no. 1 (January 2009): 70–73.

The biological set-point discussion is based on the following studies, which have excellent data, although it can be quite dense:

Farias, M. M., A. M. Cuevas, and F. Rodriguez. "Set-Point Theory and Obesity." *Metabolic Syndrome and Related Disorders* 9, no. 2 (April 2011): 85–89.

Müller, M. J., A. Bosy-Westphal, and S. B. Heymsfield. "Is There Evidence for a Set Point That Regulates Human Body Weight?" *F1000 Medicine Report* 2 (August 9, 2010): 59.

I provided the basic information about genetics in this chapter by summarizing the following studies:

Farooqi, S., and S. O'Rahilly. "Genetics of Obesity in Humans." *Endocrine Reviews* 27, no. 7 (December 2006): 710–718.

Herrera, B. M., S. Keildson, and C. M. Lindgren. "Genetics and Epigenetics of Obesity." *Maturitas* 69, no. 1 (May 2011): 41–49.

Ramachandrappa, S., and I. S. Farooqi. "Genetic Approaches to Understanding Human Obesity." *Journal of Clinical Investigation* 121, no. 6 (June 2011): 2080–2086.

I referenced studies showing the relationship between doctors and patients.

The discussion on artificial sweeteners and soda is based on studies conducted in the last ten years. It may not be well known by the public, but the scientific community has been doing research on this for more than a decade. The following studies served as the basis for the discussion in the chapter:

Elfhag, K., P. Tynelius, and F. Rasmussen. "Sugar-Sweetened and Artificially Sweetened Soft Drinks in Association to Restrained, External and Emotional Eating." *Physiology and Behavior* 91, no. 2–3 (2007): 191–195.

Green, E., and C. Murphy. "Altered Processing of Sweet Taste in the Brain of Diet Soda Drinkers." *Physiology and Behavior* (May 11, 2012).

Mahar, A., and L. M. Duizer. "The Effect of Frequency of Consumption of Artificial Sweeteners on Sweetness Liking by Women." *Journal of Food Science* 72, no. 9 (November 2007): S714–S718.

Nettleton, J. A., P. L. Lutsey, Y. Wang, J. A. Lima, E. D. Michos, and D. R. Jacobs Jr. "Diet Soda Intake and Risk of Incident Metabolic Syndrome and Type 2 Diabetes in the Multi-Ethnic Study of Atherosclerosis (MESA)." *Diabetes Care* 32 (2009): 688–694.

The references I used for the changes in brain imaging are indeed fascinating:

Frank, G. K., T. A. Oberndorfer, A. N. Simmons, M. P. Paulus, J. L. Fudge, T. T. Yang, and W. H. Kaye. "Sucrose Activates Human Taste Pathways Differently from Artificial Sweetener." *Neuroimage* 39, no. 4 (February 15, 2008): 1559–1569.

Rudenga, K. J., and D. M. Small. "Amygdala Response to Sucrose Consumption Is Inversely Related to Artificial Sweetener Use." *Appetite* 58, no. 2 (April 2012): 504–507.

There is a vast body of literature on leptin and ghrelin. The discussion of these substances as well as neuropeptide Y is based on the following key studies:

Cummings, D. E., D. S. Weigle, S. Frayo, et al. "Plasma Ghrelin Levels after Diet-Induced Weight Loss or Gastric Bypass Surgery." *New England Journal of Medicine* 346 (2002): 1623–1630.

Rosenbaum, M., J. Hirsch, D. A. Gallagher, and R. L. Leibel. "Long-Term Persistence of Adaptive Thermogenesis in Subjects Who Have Maintained a Reduced Body Weight." *American Journal of Clinical Nutrition* 88 (2008): 906–912.

Sumithran, M. B. P., L. A. Prendergast, E. Delbridge, K. Purcell, A. Shulkes, A. Kriketos, and J. Proietto. "Long-Term Persistence of Hormonal Adaptations to Weight Loss." *New England Journal of Medicine* 365 (2011): 1597–1600.

5. Dealing with Emotional Eating and Cravings

Much of the information I reviewed on the mind and body's relationship with food, especially emotional eating, can be found in key studies such as the following:

Bryant, E. J., N. A. King, and J. E. Blundell. "Disinhibition: Its Effects on Appetite and Weight Regulation." *Obesity Reviews* 9, no. 5 (September 2008): 409–419.

Hays, N. P., and S. B. Roberts. "Aspects of Eating Behaviors 'Disinhibition' and 'Restraint' Are Related to Weight Gain and BMI in Women." *Obesity* 16, no. 1 (January 2008): 52–58.

Koenders, P. G., and T. van Strien. "Emotional Eating, Rather Than Lifestyle Behavior, Drives Weight Gain in a Prospective Study in 1562 Employees." *Journal of Occupational and Environmental Medicine* 53, no. 11 (November 2011): 1287–1293.

There is a wealth of data on the relationship between stress and obesity. I based much of the discussion in this chapter on some of the most interesting studies:

Adam, T. C., and E. S. Epel. "Stress, Eating and the Reward System." *Physiology and Behavior* 91, no. 4 (July 24, 2007): 449–458.

Torres, S. J., and C. A. Nowson. "Relationship between Stress, Eating Behavior, and Obesity." *Nutrition* 23, no. 11–12 (November–December 2007): 887–894.

In recent years, we have gained a greater appreciation of the addictive nature of some foods. Much of the discussion on this topic is based on some key research studies, including the following:

Barry, D., M. Clarke, and N. M. Petry. "Obesity and Its Relationship to Addictions: Is Overeating a Form of Addictive Behavior?" *American Journal of Addiction* 18, no. 6 (November–December 2009): 439–451.

Corsica, J. A., and M. L. Pelchat. "Food Addiction: True or False?" *Current Opinion in Gastroenterology* 26, no. 2 (March 2010): 165–169.

Gardner, E. L. "Addiction and Brain Reward and Antireward Pathways." *Advances in Psychosomatic Medicine* 30 (2011): 22–60.

Liu, Y., K. M. von Deneen, F. H. Kobeissy, and M. S. Gold. "Food Addiction and Obesity: Evidence from Bench to Bedside." *Journal of Psychoactive Drugs* 42, no. 2 (June 2010): 133–145.

Meule, A., and A. Kübler. "Food Cravings in Food Addiction: The Distinct Role of Positive Reinforcement." *Eating Behavior* 13, no. 3 (August 2012): 252–255.

Von Deneen, K. M. and Y. Liu. "Obesity as an Addiction: Why Do the Obese Eat More?" *Maturitas* 68, no. 4 (April 2011): 342–345.

I consulted some recent imaging studies. The following clearly demonstrated the findings I cited: Zhang, Y., K. M. von Deneen, J. Tian, M. S. Gold, and Y. Liu. "Food Addiction and Neuroimaging." *Current Pharmaceutical Design* 17, no. 12 (2011): 1149–1157.

The discussion on changing habits is based largely on two recent studies:

Lally, P., C. H. M. van Jaarsveld, H. W. W. Potts, and J. Wardle. "How Are Habits Formed: Modeling Habit Formation in the Real World." *European Journal of Social Psychology* 40 (2010): 998–1009.

Lally, P., J. Wardle, and B. Gardner. "Experiences of Habit Formation: A Qualitative Study." *Psychology, Health, and Medicine* 16, no. 4 (August 2011): 484–489.

It is only within the last few years that we have gained an understanding of the effect of sleep on weight. This chapter's discussion of sleep is based on the following research:

Gangwisch, J. E., D. Malaspina, B. Boden-Albala, and S. B. Heymsfield. "Inadequate Sleep as a Risk Factor for Obesity: Analyses of the NHANES I." *Sleep* 28, no. 10 October 2005): 1289–1296.

Marshall, N. S., N. Glozier, and R. R. Grunstein. "Is Sleep Duration Related to Obesity? A Critical Review of the Epidemiological Evidence." *Sleep Medicine Reviews* 12, no. 4 (August 2008): 289–298.

Patel, S. R. "Reduced Sleep as an Obesity Risk Factor." *Obesity Reviews* 10, no. 2 (November 2009): 61–68.

6. The AARP New American Diet Guidelines

In this chapter, I have focused primarily on the data for weight loss. The data related to food and diseases such as cancer, diabetes, and heart disease are found in chapter 9.

Some of the data regarding the Mediterranean diet and weight can be found in the following studies:

Shai, I., D. Schwarzfuchs, Y. Henkin, D. R. Shahar, S. Witkow, I. Greenberg, R. Golan, et al. "Dietary Intervention Randomized Controlled

Trial (DIRECT) Group: Weight Loss with a Low-Carbohydrate, Mediterranean, or Low-Fat Diet." *New England Journal of Medicine* 359, no. 3 (July 17, 2008): 229–241.

Weickert, M. O. "What Dietary Modification Best Improves Insulin Sensitivity and Why?" *Clinical Endocrinology* (May 29, 2012).

Regarding whole grains and weight, the following studies guided the recommendations:

Giacco, R., G. Della Pepa, D. Luongo, and G. Riccardi. "Whole Grain Intake in Relation to Body Weight: From Epidemiological Evidence to Clinical Trials." *Nutrition, Metabolism, and Cardiovascular Diseases* 21, no. 12 (December 2011): 901–908.

Kristensen, M., S. Toubro, M. G. Jensen, A. B. Ross, G. Riboldi, M. Petronio, S. Bügel, I. Tetens, and A. Astrup. "Whole Grain Compared with Refined Wheat Decreases the Percentage of Body Fat Following a 12-Week, Energy-Restricted Dietary Intervention in Postmenopausal Women." *Journal of Nutrition* 142, no. 4 (April 2012): 710–716.

Maki, K. C., J. M. Beiseigel, S. S. Jonnalagadda, C. K. Gugger, M. S. Reeves, M. V. Farmer, V. N. Kaden, and T. M. Rains. "Whole-Grain Ready-to-Eat Oat Cereal, as Part of a Dietary Program for Weight Loss, Reduces Low-Density Lipoprotein Cholesterol in Adults with Overweight and Obesity More Than a Dietary Program Including Low-Fiber Control Foods." *Journal of the American Dietetic Association* 110, no. 2 (February 2010): 205–214.

O'Neil, C. E., M. Zanovec, S. S. Cho, and T. A. Nicklas. "Whole Grain and Fiber Consumption Are Associated with Lower Body Weight Measures in US Adults: National Health and Nutrition Examination Survey, 1999–2004." *Nutrition Research* 30, no. 12 (December 2010): 815–822.

Ye, E. Q., S. A. Chacko, E. L. Chou, M. Kugizaki, and S. Liu. "Greater Whole-Grain Intake Is Associated with Lower Risk of Type 2 Diabetes, Cardiovascular Disease, and Weight Gain." *Journal of Nutrition* (May 30, 2012).

The recommendations on avoiding meals prepared outside the home are based on the following scientific evidence:

Bezerra's recent review showing an association between eating out of home and body weight. *Nutrition Reviews* 70, no. 2 (February 2012): 65–79.

Lachat, C., E. Nago, R. Verstraeten, D. Roberfroid, J. Van Camp, and P. Kolsteren. "Eating out of Home and Its Association with Dietary

Intake: A Systematic Review of the Evidence." *Obesity Reviews* 13, no. 4 (April 2012): 329–346.

The data on dairy and weight loss are well documented but not well known. I based the discussion and the recommendations on the following key studies:

Josse, A. R., S. A. Atkinson, M. A. Tarnopolsky, and S. M. Phillips. "Increased Consumption of Dairy Foods and Protein during Diet- and Exercise-Induced Weight Loss Promotes Fat Mass Loss and Lean Mass Gain in Overweight and Obese Premenopausal Women." *Journal of Nutrition* 141, no. 9 (September 2011): 1626–1634.

Zemel, M. B. "Role of Calcium and Dairy Products in Energy Partitioning and Weight Management." *American Journal of Clinical Nutrition* 79, no. 5 (May 2004): 907–912S.

Zemel, M. B. "The Role of Dairy Foods in Weight Management." *Journal of the American College of Nutrition* 24, no. 6 (December 2005): 537–546S.

The role of water consumption and weight loss has been studied for years, with the overwhelming amount of data showing that proper and adequate water consumption leads to weight loss. The chapter discussion is based on these key studies:

Davy, B. M., E. A. Dennis, A. L. Dengo, K. L. Wilson, and K. P. Davy. "Water Consumption Reduces Energy Intake at a Breakfast Meal in Obese Older Adults." *Journal of the American Dietetic Association* 108, no. 7 (July 2008): 1236–1239.

Dennis, E. A., A. L. Dengo, D. L. Comber, K. D. Flack, J. Savla, K. P. Davy, and B. M. Davy. "Water Consumption Increases Weight Loss during a Hypocaloric Diet Intervention in Middle-Aged and Older Adults." *Obesity* 18, no. 2 (February 2010): 300–307.

Van Walleghen, E. L., J. S. Orr, C. L. Gentile, and B. M. Davy. "Premeal Water Consumption Reduces Meal Energy Intake in Older but Not Younger Subjects." *Obesity* 15 (January 2001): 93–99.

I noted that some of the strongest data relate to the need to eat breakfast in order to lose weight. This was based on the following research:

Deshmukh-Taskar, P. R., T. A. Nicklas, C. E. O'Neil, D. R. Keast, J. D. Radcliffe, and S. Cho. "The Relationship of Breakfast Skipping and Type of Breakfast Consumption with Nutrient Intake and Weight Status in Children and Adolescents: The National Health and Nutrition Examination Survey, 1999–2006." *Journal of the American Dietetic Association* 110, no. 6 (June 2010): 869–878.

Song, W. O., O. K. Chun, S. Obayashi, S. Cho, and C. E. Chung. "Is Consumption of Breakfast Associated with Body Mass Index in US Adults?" *Journal of the American Dietetic Association* 105, no. 9 (September 2005): 1373–1382.

Wyatt, H. R., G. K. Grunwald, C. L. Mosca, M. L. Klem, R. R. Wing, and J. O Hill. "Long-Term Weight Loss and Breakfast in Subjects in the National Weight Control Registry." *Obesity Research* 10, no. 2 (February 2002): 78–82.

The CDC reports on a bread as the number one source of sodium. It also details other sources of sodium. Moshfegh, A. J., et al. "Vital Signs: Food Categories Contributing the Most to Sodium Consumption—United States, 2007–2008." *Morbidity and Mortality Weekly Report* 61 (2012).

9. Reducing Your Risk of Disease: Cancer, Heart Disease, and Diabetes

As I noted throughout the book, what we eat has a profound influence on whether we develop certain diseases. The discussion and recommendations on nutrition and cancer are largely based on the NIH-AARP Diet and Health Study. My friend and colleague Dr. Albert Hollenbeck has been a principal investigator of the study. I worked on distilling the information from the following studies down to the relevant points discussed in this chapter. (Normally, I would not include this many references in this format, but given the importance of the information, I wanted it to be available to you.)

Aschebrook-Kilfoy, B., A. J. Cross, R. Z. Stolzenberg-Solomon, A. Schatzkin, A. R. Hollenbeck, R. Sinha, and M. H. Ward. "Pancreatic Cancer and Exposure to Dietary Nitrate and Nitrite in the NIH-AARP Diet and Health Study." *American Journal of Epidemiology* 174, no. 3 (August 1, 2011): 305–315.

Aschebrook-Kilfoy, B., M. H. Ward, G. L. Gierach, A. Schatzkin, A. R. Hollenbeck, R. Sinha, and A. J. Cross. "Epithelial Ovarian Cancer and Exposure to Dietary Nitrate and Nitrite in the NIH-AARP Diet and Health Study." *European Journal of Cancer Prevention* 21, no. 1 (January 2012): 65–72.

Blank, M. M., N. Wentzensen, M. A. Murphy, A. Hollenbeck, and Y. Park. "Dietary Fat Intake and Risk of Ovarian Cancer in the NIH-AARP Diet and Health Study." *British Journal of Cancer* 106, no. 3 (January 31, 2012): 596–602.

Davies, N. J., L. Batehup, and. Thomas. "The Role of Diet and Physical Activity in Breast, Colorectal, and Prostate Cancer Survivorship: A Review of the Literature." *British Journal of Cancer* 105, no. 1 (November 8, 2011): S52–S73.

Ferrucci, L. M., R. Sinha, M. H. Ward, B. I. Graubard, A. R. Hollenbeck, B. A. Kilfoy, A. Schatzkin, D. S. Michaud, and A. J. Cross. "Meat and Components of Meat and the Risk of Bladder Cancer in the NIH-AARP Diet and Health Study." *Cancer* 116, no. 18 (September 15, 2010): 4345–4353.

Freedman, N. D., Y. Park, A. F. Subar, A. R. Hollenbeck, M. F. Leitzmann, A. Schatzkin, and C. C. Abnet. "Fruit and Vegetable Intake and Head and Neck Cancer Risk in a Large United States Prospective Cohort Study." *International Journal of Cancer* 122, no. 10 (May 15, 2008): 2330–2336.

George, S. M., S. C. Moore, W. H. Chow, A. Schatzkin, A. R. Hollenbeck, and C. E. Matthews. "A Prospective Analysis of Prolonged Sitting Time and Risk of Renal Cell Carcinoma among 300,000 Older Adults." *Annals of Epidemiology* 21, no. 10 (October 2011): 787–790.

La Vecchia, C. "Mediterranean Diet and Cancer." *Public Health Nutrition* 7, no. 7 (October 2004): 965–968.

Lew, J. Q., W. H. Chow, A. R. Hollenbeck, A. Schatzkin, and Y. Park. "Alcohol Consumption and Risk of Renal Cell Cancer: The NIH-AARP Diet and Health Study." *British Journal of Cancer* 104, no. 3 (February 1, 2011): 537–541.

Mitrou, P. N., V. Kipnis, A. C. Thiébaut, J. Reedy, A. F. Subar, E. Wirfält, A. Flood, et al. "Mediterranean Dietary Pattern and Prediction of All-Cause Mortality in a US Population: Results from the NIH-AARP Diet and Health Study." *Archives of Internal Medicine* 167, no. 22 (December 10, 2007): 2461–2468.

O'Doherty, M. G., N. D. Freedman, A. R. Hollenbeck, A. Schatzkin, L. J. Murray, M. M. Cantwell, and C. C. Abnet. "Association of Dietary Fat Intakes with Risk of Esophageal and Gastric Cancer in the NIH-AARP Diet and Health Study." *International Journal of Cancer* (November 24, 2011).

Park, Y., L. A. Brinton, A. F. Subar, A. Hollenbeck, and A. Schatzkin. "Dietary Fiber Intake and Risk of Breast Cancer in Postmenopausal Women: The National Institutes of Health-AARP Diet and Health Study." *American Journal of Clinical Nutrition* 90, no. 3 (September 2009): 664–671.

Schatzkin, A., T. Mouw, Y. Park, A. F. Subar, V. Kipnis, A. Hollenbeck, M. F. Leitzmann, and F. E. Thompson. "Dietary Fiber and Whole-Grain Consumption in Relation to Colorectal Cancer in the NIH-AARP Diet and Health Study." *American Journal of Clinical Nutrition* 85, no. 5 (May 2007): 1353–1360.

Thiébaut, A. C., V. Chajès, M. Gerber, M. C. Boutron-Ruault, V. Joulin, G. Lenoir, F. Berrino, E. Riboli, J. Bénichou, and F. Clavel-Chapelon. "Dietary Intakes of Omega-6 and Omega-3 Polyunsaturated Fatty Acids and the Risk of Breast Cancer." *International Journal of Cancer* 124, no. 4 (February 15, 2009): 924–931.

Thiébaut, A. C., L. Jiao, D. T. Silverman, A. J. Cross, F. E. Thompson, A. F. Subar, A. R. Hollenbeck, A. Schatzkin, and R. Z. Stolzenberg-Solomon. "Dietary Fatty Acids and Pancreatic Cancer in the NIH-AARP Diet and Health Study." *Journal of the National Cancer Institute* 101, no. 14 (July 15, 2009): 1001–1011.

In this chapter, I discussed the relationship between meat and cancer. I have included some key references that are good resources for additional information:

John, E. M., M. C. Stern, R. Sinha, and J. Koo. "Meat Consumption, Cooking Practices, Meat Mutagens, and Risk of Prostate Cancer." *Nutrition and Cancer* 63, no. 4 (2011): 525–537.

Major, J. M., A. J. Cross, J. L. Watters, A. R. Hollenbeck, B. I. Graubard, and R. Sinha. "Patterns of Meat Intake and Risk of Prostate Cancer among African-Americans in a Large Prospective Study." *Cancer Causes and Control* 22, no. 12 (December 2011): 1691–1698.

Numerous studies relate to alcohol consumption and cancer. Several have already been referenced. Two additional ones that help to serve as a basis for the recommendations in the book are the following:

Chen, W. Y., B. Rosner, S. E. Hankinson, G. A. Colditz, and W. C. Willett. "Moderate Alcohol Consumption during Adult Life, Drinking Patterns, and Breast Cancer Risk." *Journal of the American Medical Association* 306, no. 17 (November 2, 2011): 1884–1890.

Crockett, S. D., M. D. Long, E. S. Dellon, C. F. Martin, J. A. Galanko, and R. S. Sandler. "Inverse Relationship between Moderate Alcohol Intake and Rectal Cancer: Analysis of the North Carolina Colon Cancer Study." *Diseases of the Colon and Rectum* 54, no. 7 (July 2011): 887–894.

The studies relating to coffee and health have been consistent over time in showing a health benefit. Again, the NIH-AARP Study helped to provide the best guidance. Its most recent study was reported this year in Freedman, N. D., Y. Park, C. C. Abnet, A. R. Hollenbeck, and R. Sinha. "Association of Coffee Drinking with Total and Cause-Specific Mortality." *New England Journal of Medicine* 366, no. 20 (May 17, 2012): 1891–1904.

Other studies include the following:

Ganmaa, D., W. C. Willett, T. Y. Li, D. Feskanich, R. M. van Dam, E. Lopez-Garcia, D. J. Hunter, and M. D. Holmes. "Coffee, Tea, Caffeine and Risk of Breast Cancer: A 22-Year Follow-Up." *International Journal of Cancer* 122, no. 9 (May 1, 2008): 2071–2076.

Giri, A., S. R. Sturgeon, N. Luisi, E. Bertone-Johnson, R. Balasubramanian, and K. W. Reeves. "Caffeinated Coffee, Decaffeinated Coffee and Endometrial Cancer Risk: A Prospective Cohort Study among US Postmenopausal Women." *Nutrients* 3, no. 11 (November 2011): 937–950.

Lopez-Garcia, E., R. M. van Dam, T. Y. Li, F. Rodriguez-Artalejo, and F. B. Hu. "The Relationship of Coffee Consumption with Mortality." *Annals of Internal Medicine* 148, no. 12 (June 17, 2008): 904–914.

Van Dam, R. M., and F. B. Hu. "Coffee Consumption and Risk of Type 2 Diabetes: A Systematic Review." *Journal of the American Medical Association* 294, no. 1 (July 2005): 97–104.

Wilson, K. M., J. L. Kasperzyk, J. R. Rider, S. Kenfield, R. M. van Dam, M. J. Stampfer, E. Giovannucci, and L. A. Mucci. "Coffee Consumption and Prostate Cancer Risk and Progression in the Health Professionals Follow-Up Study." *Journal of the National Cancer Institute* 103, no. 11 (June 8, 2011): 876–884.

Much of what we know about diet and heart disease has been guided by the following key studies:

Hung, H. C., K. J. Joshipura, R. Jiang, F. B. Hu, D. Hunter, S. A. Smith-Warner, G. A. Colditz, B. Rosner, D. Spiegelman, and W. C. Willett. "Fruit and Vegetable Intake and Risk of Major Chronic Disease." *Journal of the National Cancer Institute* 96, no. 21 (November 3, 2004): 1577–1584.

Mozaffarian, D., and J. H. Wu. "Omega-3 Fatty Acids and Cardiovascular Disease: Effects on Risk Factors, Molecular Pathways, and Clinical Events." *Journal of the American College of Cardiology* 58, no. 20 (November 8, 2011): 2047–2067.

There are numerous well-designed studies on the relationship between cholesterol (both blood and dietary) on heart disease. Some of the studies I used to provide guidance in this chapter are the following:

Huxley, R., S. Lewington, and R. Clarke. "Cholesterol, Coronary Heart Disease and Stroke: A Review of Published Evidence from Observational Studies and Randomized Controlled Trials." *Seminars in Vascular Medicine* 2, no. 3 (August 2002): 315–323.

Jakobsen, M. U., E. J. O'Reilly, B. L. Heitmann, M. A. Pereira, K. Bälter, G. E. Fraser, U. Goldbourt, et al. "Major Types of Dietary Fat and Risk of Coronary Heart Disease: A Pooled Analysis of 11 Cohort Studies." *American Journal of Clinical Nutrition* 89, no. 5 (May 2009): 1425–1432.

Willett, W. C. "Dietary Fats and Coronary Heart Disease." *Journal of Internal Medicine* (May 14, 2012).

The discussion on soda and heart disease in this chapter is based on two very recent and well-designed studies:

De Koning, L. "Sweetened Beverage Consumption, Incident Coronary Heart Disease, and Biomarkers of Risk in Men." *Circulation* 125, no. 14 (April 10, 2012): 1735–1741.

Stanhope, K. L. "Consumption of Fructose and High-Fructose Corn Syrup Increase Postprandial Triglycerides, LDL-Cholesterol, and Apolipoprotein B in Young Men and Women." *Journal of Clinical Endocrinology and Metabolism* (2011).

The specific data on red meat and increased mortality can be found in Pan, A., Q. Sun, A. M. Bernstein, M. B. Schulze, J. E. Manson, M. J. Stampfer, W. C. Willett, and F. B. Hu. "Red Meat Consumption and Mortality: Results from 2 Prospective Cohort Studies." *Archives of Internal Medicine* 172, no. 7 (April 9, 2012): 555–563. My good friend Dr. Dean Ornish has an excellent commentary on the article in the same issue. He too proposes the concept of "what you include is as important as what you exclude" in obtaining and maintaining good health.

I included more data on alcohol—specifically its relationship to heart disease. This research continues to evolve, but the key studies used to guide recommendations in this chapter include the following:

Brien, S. E., P. E. Ronksley, B. J. Turner, K. J. Mukamal, and W. A. Ghali. "Effect of Alcohol Consumption on Biological Markers Associated with Risk of Coronary Heart Disease: Systematic Review and Meta-Analysis of Interventional Studies." *British Medical Journal* (February 22, 2011).

Jimenez, M., S. E. Chiuve, R. J. Glynn, M. J. Stampfer, C. A. Camargo Jr., W. C. Willett, J. E. Manson, and K. M. Rexrode. "Alcohol Consumption and Risk of Stroke in Women." *Stroke* 43, no. 4 (April 2012): 939–945.

Roerecke, M., and J. Rehm. "The Cardioprotective Association of Average Alcohol Consumption and Ischaemic Heart Disease: A Systematic Review and Meta-Analysis." *Addiction* 107, no. 7 (July 2012): 1246–1260.

The data on dark chocolate protecting the heart are pretty convincing. The recommendations in this chapter are based on the following studies:

Buitrago-Lopez, A., J. Sanderson, L. Johnson, S. Warnakula, A. Wood, E. Di Angelantonio, and O. H. Franco. "Chocolate Consumption and Cardiometabolic Disorders: Systematic Review and Meta-Analysis." *British Medical Journal* (August 26, 2011).

Djoussé, L., P. N. Hopkins, K. E. North, J. S. Pankow, D. K. Arnett, and R. C. Ellison. "Chocolate Consumption Is Inversely Associated with Prevalent Coronary Heart Disease: The National Heart, Lung, and Blood Institute Family Heart Study." *Clinical Nutrition* 30, no. 2 (April 2011): 182–187.

Khawaja, O., J. M. Gaziano, and L. Djoussé. "Chocolate and Coronary Heart Disease: A Systematic Review." *Current Atherosclerosis Reports* 13, no. 6 (December 2011): 447–452.

Zomer, E., A. Owen, D. J. Magliano, D. Liew, and C. M. Reid. "The Effectiveness and Cost Effectiveness of Dark Chocolate Consumption as Prevention Therapy in People at High Risk of Cardiovascular Disease: Best Case Scenario Analysis Using a Markov Model." *British Journal of Medicine* (May 30, 2012).

The relation between diet and diabetes has been studied for decades, and good data support the recommendations in this chapter. The following studies helped to clarify the recent and relevant information:

Lazarou, C., D. Panagiotakos, and A. L. Matalas. "The Role of Diet in Prevention and Management of Type 2 Diabetes: Implications for Public Health." *Critical Reviews in Food Science and Nutrition* 52, no. 5 (2012): 382–389.

Männistö, S., J. Kontto, M. Kataja-Tuomola, D. Albanes, and J. Virtamo. "High Processed Meat Consumption Is a Risk Factor of Type 2 Diabetes in the Alpha-Tocopherol, Beta-Carotene Cancer Prevention Study." *British Journal of Nutrition* (June 2010).

Salas-Salvadó, J., M. A. Martinez-González, M. Bulló, and E. Ros. "The Role of Diet in the Prevention of Type 2 Diabetes." *Nutrition, Metabolism, and Cardiovascular Diseases* 21, no. 2 (September 2011): B32–48.

10. Eat Well, Get Fit, Sharpen Your Brain

The relationship between exercise and longevity is well documented. The findings from the following studies guided the recommendations in this chapter:

Dumurgier, J., F. Crivello, B. Mazoyer, I. Ahmed, B. Tavernier, D. Grabli, C. François, N. Tzourio-Mazoyer, C. Tzourio, and A. Elbaz. "MRI Atrophy of the Caudate Nucleus and Slower Walking Speed in the Elderly." *Neuroimage* 60, no. 2 (April 2, 2012): 871–878.

Lee, I. M., C. C. Hsieh, and R. S. Paffenbarger Jr. "Exercise Intensity and Longevity in Men: The Harvard Alumni Health Study." *Journal of the American Medical Association* 273, no. 15 (April 19, 1995): 1179–1184.

Lee, I. M., K. M. Rexrode, N. R. Cook, J. E. Manson, and J. E. Buring. "Physical Activity and Coronary Heart Disease in Women: Is 'No Pain, No Gain' Passé?" *Journal of the American Medical Association* 285, no. 11 (March 21, 2001): 1447–1454.

I discussed earlier the importance of sleep in losing weight. In this chapter, I discussed how sleep affects longevity. An excellent review of the current thinking on how sleep affects life span is Cappuccio, F. P., L. D'Elia, P. Strazzullo, and M. A. Miller. "Sleep Duration and All-Cause Mortality: A Systematic Review and Meta-Analysis of Prospective Studies." *Sleep* 33, no. 5 (May 2010): 585–592.

The information relating to positive attitude as well as optimism and longevity is based on the following good science:

Kato, K., R. Zweig, N. Barzilai, and G. Atzmon. "Positive Attitude towards Life and Emotional Expression as Personality Phenotypes for Centenarians." *Aging* (May 21, 2012).

Martin, P., J. Baenziger, M. Macdonald, I. C. Siegler, and L. W. Poon. "Engaged Lifestyle, Personality, and Mental Status among Centenarians." *Journal of Adult Development* 16, no. 4 (December 2009): 199–208.

Rasmussen, H. N., M. F. Scheier, and J. B. Greenhouse. "Optimism and Physical Health: A Meta-Analytic Review." *Annals of Behavioral Medicine* 37, no. 3 (June 2009): 239–256.

The data on diet and healthy brains continue to evolve. The recommendations are based on the following studies:

Gelber, R. P., H. Petrovitch, K. H. Masaki, G. W. Ross, and L. R. White. "Coffee Intake in Midlife and Risk of Dementia and Its Neuropathologic Correlates." *Journal of Alzheimer's Disease* 23, no. 4 (2011): 607–615.

Gu, Y., J. W. Nieves, Y. Stern, J. A. Luchsinger, and N. Scarmeas. "Food Combination and Alzheimer Disease Risk: A Protective Diet." *Archives of Neurology* 67, no. 6 (June 2010): 699–706.

Scarmeas, N., J. A. Luchsinger, N. Schupf, A. M. Brickman, S. Cosentino, M. X. Tang, and Y. Stern. "Physical Activity, Diet, and Risk of Alzheimer Disease." *Journal of the American Medical Association* 302, no. 6 (August 12, 2009): 627–637.

Solfrizzi, V., F. Panza, V. Frisardi, D. Seripa, G. Logroscino, B. P. Imbimbo, and A. Pilotto. "Diet and Alzheimer's Disease Risk Factors or Prevention: The Current Evidence." *Expert Review of Neurotherapeutics* 11, no. 5 (May 2011): 677–708.

Resources

The AARP website (www.aarp.org) and Discovery Channel (www .discoverychannelpatiented.com) have a wealth of additional resources for you to learn more about healthy eating, exercising, and living longer. I have included some additional websites here that I think you might be interested in checking out.

AARP, www.AARP.org. AARP's website features a full suite of health- and diet-related tools, articles, and recipes. AARP.org/healthtools offers a Body Mass Index (BMI) Calculator, Drug Interaction Checker, and Health Encyclopedia, among other interactive tools. AARP.org/health provides articles about fitness, diet, and medical discoveries. AARP.org/food is home to healthy and fun menu options and recipes, including recipes for a variety of specialized dietary needs. The AARP website also includes health- and dining-related discount offers for AARP members. (Full membership to AARP is available to people over fifty and costs $16 a year.) Much information is available in Spanish.

Discovery Fit and Health, www.health.discovery.com. Discovery is an online resource for health, fitness, and wellness information. There are many videos on healthy eating, answers to common health questions, and a demonstration of different exercises that people of all ages can do. There are also numerous interactive games to teach you the latest health information and then test you on it in a fun and exciting way. Be sure to check out the blogs of some of the most well-known nutrition and fitness experts in the world.

Academy of Nutrition and Dietetics, www.eatright.org. As the world's largest organization of food and nutrition professionals, the academy provides nutrition information to health professionals and the general public. Click on the Public tab to access content on home food safety, food allergies, and a nutrition reading list. The Tip of the Day and the Question of the Day will regularly satisfy your nutrition-related curiosities. For the tech-savvy crowd, there are reviews of weight-management apps. There is also an excellent section that reviews many popular diets. The Top Searches feature is a great way to see what other users are searching for.

Choose My Plate, www.choosemyplate.gov/. This site provides numerous resources to help the public make wise dietary choices and eat in accordance with the federal government's My Plate guidelines. One outstanding tool is the Super Tracker, which allows you to plan, analyze, and track your diet and physical activity. The Calorie Burn Chart reveals how many calories you may actually be burning while doing your routine activities, and the Empty Calories Chart shows you where extra calories may have been sneaking into your diet.

Let's Move! www.letsmove.gov/. This government initiative strives to promote greater physical activity among youth. The family- and community-focused approach is perfect for those who are looking to achieve a healthier life along with a spouse or children. The website is formatted with tabs for tips on healthy eating and active lifestyle steps. The Eat Healthy tab contains a helpful Gardening Guide that takes the trepidation out of growing your own fresh produce. Check out the Take Action tab for tools to promote health and nutrition on a larger scale to schools and public officials.

Mediterranean Food Alliance, http://oldwayspt.org/programs/mediterranean-foods-alliance. This program by Oldways aims to increase consumer awareness of the Mediterranean diet. An excellent resource here is the Shopping, Cooking, and Eating section, which serves as a guide to stocking your kitchen Mediterranean-style. You will find tips on choosing the right cooking equipment, maintaining portion control, and sticking to your diet even at parties. Also check out National Mediterranean Diet Month and the Mediterranean food pyramid.

Nutrition.gov, www.nutrition.gov/. Brought to you by the National Agricultural Library, this government resource seeks to provide easy online access to food and nutrition information. A great feature here is the Know Your Farmer, Know Your Food project, which aims to promote responsible purchasing of locally farmed foods. Browse the Spotlights section for fresh content, like recipes and top ten lists. You can also find governmental dietary guidelines, fact sheets about dietary supplements, information on food safety, and much more. Registered dietitians are there to help you from the Contact Us page. The full site is also available in Spanish.

President's Council on Fitness, Sports, and Nutrition, www.fitness .gov/. Remember the president's fitness challenge when you were in grade school? It's still around! This committee of volunteer citizens advises the government on healthy and active lifestyles. A great resource here is the Fit Facts and Tips section, where you can find useful facts and tips on exercise, nutrition, fitness for expectant mothers, and more. You can also find the federal guidelines for diet and exercise to make sure you're meeting national health goals and staying a cut above the rest. Take a moment to read the President's Challenge and the President's Active Lifestyle Award.

Shape Up America, www.shapeup.org. This nonprofit organization is dedicated to raising awareness of obesity and providing information on healthy weight management. A particularly useful tool here is the Meal Upgrade, which offers simple solutions for easy substitutions in your favorite recipes, so you can eat the foods you love and be health-conscious at the same time. Also, be sure to take a look at the Body Fat tab, which clearly explains how to measure body fat, interpret your measurements, and differentiate among the many methods of determining your body composition.

USDA National Nutrient Database, http://ndb.nal.usda.gov/. Not everything we eat comes with a nutrition label. Ever wonder what's in the meal you're eating? This database maintains dietary information on more than eight thousand food items, and the list is still growing. Simply enter what you ate and how much, and the database will return information on how many servings, calories, fats, proteins, and so on, from the food composition to the macronutrients. Not all foods are listed, especially unique international foods, but the list grows and may eventually accommodate those searches.

Index